Contents

List of Colour Illustrations

Fig. 1 Acute moist dermatitis on the gluteal region of a dog.
Fig. 2 Facial fold pyoderma in a Pekingese dog.
Fig. 3 Vulvar fold pyoderma in a bulldog.
Fig. 4 Papules and pustules in the glabrous skin of the ventral abdomen of a dog with superficial pyoderma.
Fig. 5 Crusting lesion of superficial pyoderma in a dog.
Fig. 6 Epidermal collarette lesion of superficial pyoderma (courtesy M. Geary).
Fig. 7 Lesions of canine acne (courtesy I.S. Mason).
Fig. 8 Nasal pyoderma in a dog.
Fig. 9 Same dog as in Fig. 8 after treatment with potentiated sulphonamide for 3 weeks.
Fig. 10 Callus pyoderma on the elbow of a Great Dane.
Fig. 11 Generalized deep pyoderma of the thorax and forelimb of an Irish setter.
Fig. 12 Feline pyoderma in the neck region (cat-bite sepsis).
Fig. 13 Chronic flea-bite hypersensitivity in a Labrador dog.
Fig. 14 Bilaterally symmetrical alopecia in a cat due to flea-bite hypersensitivity.
Fig. 15 *Cheyletiella* sp. (courtesy M. Geary).
Fig. 16 Excessive scale in a spaniel due to *Cheyletiella* infestation.
Fig. 17 Extensive alopecia and pruritic lesions in a cat with *Cheyletiella* infestation.
Fig. 18 *Cheyletiella* eggs attached to cat hairs (courtesy Mike Caygill).
Fig. 19 *Sarcoptes scabiei* var. *canis*.
Fig. 20 Severe lesions of scabies in a cocker spaniel.
Fig. 21 *Demodex canis*.
Fig. 22 Localized demodicosis in a dog.
Fig. 23 Generalized squamous demodicosis in a Jack Russell terrier.
Fig. 24 Demodicosis in a 9-year-old Dobermann pinscher. The dog developed osteosarcoma of the ilium 2 months after onset of the demodicosis.
Fig. 25 Generalized demodicosis with secondary pyoderma in a 9-month-old crossbred dog.
Fig. 26 Same dog as in Fig. 25 4 months after treatment with Amitraz and antibacterial agents.
Fig. 27 *Demodex cati* (courtesy D. Scarff).
Fig. 28 Unnamed *Demodex* sp. of the cat (courtesy C. Chesney).
Fig. 29 *Otodectes cynotis*.
Fig. 30 Erythematous facial lesions in a cat due to hypersensitivity to *Otodectes*.
Fig. 31 *Neotrombicula autumnalis* (courtesy L.R. Thomsett).
Fig. 32 Pododermatitis in a West Highland white terrier due to hypersensitivity to *Neotrombicula autumnalis* (courtesy K.L. Thoday).
Fig. 33 Ulceration and hyperkeratosis of the footpads of a dog due to hookworm larvae (courtesy K.L. Thoday).
Fig. 34 Generalized circular lesions of *Microsporum canis* in a dog.
Fig. 35 Alopecia on the thorax of a Yorkshire terrier due to *Trichophyton mentagrophytes*.
Fig. 36 Kerion lesion due to *Microsporum canis* on the chin of a German shepherd dog.
Fig. 37 *Microsporum canis* lesion in a cat.
Fig. 38 Hyperkeratosis of the footpads of a dog with distemper virus infection.
Fig. 39 Bilaterally symmetrical alopecia due to hypothyroidism in a Scottish terrier.

Skin Diseases in the
Dog and Cat

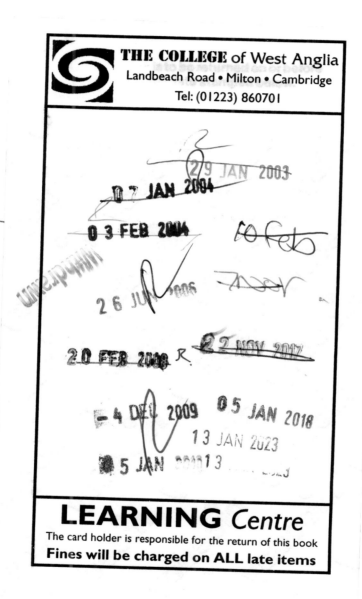

LIBRARY OF VETERINARY PRACTICE

EDITORS

C.J. PRICE MA, VetMB, MRCVS
The Veterinary Hospital
49 Cambridge Street
Aylesbury, Bucks

P.G.C. BEDFORD BVetMed, PhD, DVOphthal, FRCVS
Royal Veterinary College
Hawkshead Lane, North Mymms, Hatfield, Herts

J.B. SUTTON JP, MRCVS
2 Friarswood Road
Newcastle-under-Lyme, Staffs

LIBRARY OF VETERINARY PRACTICE

Skin Diseases in the Dog and Cat

D.I. GRANT BVetMed, Cert SAD, FRCVS

SECOND EDITION

OXFORD

BLACKWELL SCIENTIFIC PUBLICATIONS

LONDON EDINBURGH BOSTON

MELBOURNE PARIS BERLIN VIENNA

© 1986, 1991 by
Blackwell Scientific Publications
Editorial Offices:
Osney Mead, Oxford OX2 0EL
25 John Street, London WC1N 2BL
23 Ainslie Place, Edinburgh EH3 6AJ
3 Cambridge Center, Cambridge
  Massachusetts 02142, USA
54 University Street, Carlton
  Victoria 3053, Australia

Other Editorial Offices:
Arnette SA
2, rue Casimir-Delavigne
75006 Paris
France

Blackwell Wissenschaft
Meinekestrasse 4
D-1000 Berlin 15
Germany

Blackwell MZV
Feldgasse 13
A-1238 Wien
Austria

First published 1986
Second edition 1991

Set by Setrite Typesetters, Hong Kong
Printed and bound in Great Britain
at the University Press, Cambridge

DISTRIBUTORS

Marston Book Services Ltd
PO Box 87
Oxford OX2 0DT
(*Orders*: Tel: 0865 791155
         Fax: 0865 791927
         Telex: 837515)

USA
  Mosby-Year Book, Inc.
  11830 Westline Industrial Drive
  St Louis, Missouri 63146
  (*Orders*: Tel: 800 633−6699)

Canada
  Mosby-Year Book, Inc.
  5240 Finch Avenue East
  Scarborough, Ontario
  (*Orders* Tel: 416 298−1588)

Australia
  Blackwell Scientific Publications
  (Australia) Pty Ltd
  54 University Street
  Carlton, Victoria 3053
  (*Orders*: Tel: 03 347−0300)

British Library
Cataloguing in Publication Data

Grant, D.I.
  Skin diseases in the dog and the cat. —
  2nd. ed.
  1. Livestock: Dogs. Skin. Diseases
  2. Pets: Cats. Skin. Diseases
  I. Title II. Series
  636.708965

ISBN 0−632−02935−8

Colour illustrations appear between pages 118 and 119.

Preface

In writing the second edition of this book the aim has remained the same — to assist veterinary surgeons and students to learn essential facts about skin diseases in the dog and cat. It is hoped that readers will be sufficiently stimulated to study the subject further, by consulting the standard texts and suggested reading at the end of the book, and by joining specialist study groups such as the British Veterinary Dermatology Study Group and the European Society of Veterinary Dermatology.

The material has been updated and there is additional information on nail, ear and eye disease. It is hoped that readers will read the entire text in a day or so and not use the book as a reference text which it is not designed to be.

I am very grateful to the following colleagues for their help and criticism during the writing of this edition: Colin Price, Martin Briggs, David Scarff, Dr Keith Thoday and Dr Ian Mason.

D.I. GRANT
London, 1990

1/Approach to the Skin Case

GENERAL POINTS

- it is commonly stated that in an average small animal practice approximately 20% of all cases are dermatological. Some of these cases will be obvious, presenting no diagnostic difficulty, for example a pruritic dog with a heavy flea infestation
- many cases, however, need the same kind of systematic approach that would be necessary to investigate a neurological or cardio-vascular problem. It is a mistake to attempt to diagnose conditions based on the presenting lesions as many conditions appear clinically similar
- the diagnosis is best made by a careful history (most important), a general physical examination followed by a dermatological examination, and by the use of laboratory and other diagnostic techniques
- only if a diagnosis is made can logical specific treatment and an accurate prognosis be given
- in a busy small animal practice, the veterinary surgeon may feel that there is inadequate time to investigate skin cases properly; however, if potentially difficult cases are identified early, there is no reason why extra time cannot be found to undertake a detailed investigation. In the long run this will save time and money
- within any one particular practice it is useful to encourage one or more veterinary surgeons to take a special interest in dermatology, and to ensure continuity with the investigation of cases. Too many opinions with frequent changes of treatment are frustrating for the owner and usually detrimental to the animal
- also useful is the adoption of a glucocorticoid policy adhered to by all members of the practice. These valuable drugs are frequently abused, so to avoid this problem the following is suggested:
  - a short-term minimum dose initially to control symptoms prior to making a precise diagnosis
  - no long-term therapy unless specifically indicated, such as in atopy, and even then only when all other avenues of investigation have been explored to the satisfaction of both the veterinary surgeon and the owner; under these circumstances use alternate-day prednisolone (see p. 30) by mouth, not repositol gluco-corticoid injections

1

THE LOGICAL INVESTIGATION OF THE SKIN CASE

- always begin by taking a careful history
- listening skills are important, but the veterinary surgeon should not allow the owner to ramble
- the basic aim of the history is to build a picture of the disease from its beginning. An intelligent co-operative owner will frequently describe the condition classically
- note initially the owner's complaint, such as pruritus, shedding, alopecia, lesions (including any involving the owner)
- breed, as some breeds are predisposed to skin conditions, for example boxers to neoplastic conditions, English setters to atopy
- age: demodicosis in young dogs; atopy frequently starts in dogs 1 to 3 years of age; neoplasia usually in older dogs
- sex: specific gonadal problems, change of sexual behaviour, for example Sertoli's cell tumour

Specific questions

- when did the problem begin?
- what time of year? Atopy is frequently seasonal initially. Natural remission in winter?
- pruritic or non-pruritic? Pruritic problems suggest ectoparasites, hypersensitivity disorders, seborrhoea; absence of pruritus suggests endocrinopathies, and some neoplastic conditions. It is important to establish whether there was pruritus when the problem began, since secondary pyoderma may result in pruritus
- where did the lesions first appear? Canine scabies frequently begins on the pinnae, demodicosis on the head and forelimbs, and flea-bite hypersensitivity on the posterior dorsum.
- other animals affected?
- humans affected? Contagion
- when were fleas last seen? what measures were taken to control them? Fleas are frequently inadequately treated

Non-specific questions

Diet

- is the diet satisfactory? Generic dry foods may be deficient in fatty acids. Is digestion apparently normal? i.e. no vomiting, no diarrhoea and normal frequency of defaecation
- a list is made of all components of the diet including titbits. Such a list is necessary in formulating an elimination diet for the investigation of food hypersensitivity

Appetite

- increased? Diabetes mellitus, hyperadrenocorticism
- decreased? Liver, kidney disease, hypothyroidism

Thirst

- increased? Diabetes mellitus, hyperadrenocorticism, liver and kidney disease

Exercise tolerance

- lethargy is often noted with hypothyroidism
- weakness is usually a feature of hyperadrenocorticism due to muscle atrophy

Oestrus cycle

- may be absent or with abnormal intervals in hypothyroidism and hyperadrenocorticism
- may be prolonged in ovarian imbalance type 2

Respiratory signs

- sneezing is occasionally seen in atopic dogs

Other points

- a note is made of the dog's bedding and contact materials in the home, and of its general environment when out walking. This information is required for the investigation or primary irritant contact dermatitis and contact hypersensitivity
- previous treatments are noted. An initial response to glucocorticoids followed by relapse when they cease suggests a hypersensitivity disorder
- have treatments been properly administered by the owner? Shampoos are frequently inefficiently done. Ensure that instructions are clear and assess the ability to comply with instructions. It is essential to carry out treatment in the hospital if the owner cannot cope with treatment at home

PHYSICAL EXAMINATION

- the purpose of the physical examination is to detect signs of systemic disease which may be associated with or be the cause of the dermatological condition

- good lighting is essential, with magnification
- examine the entire animal. Begin at the head and work back systematically, examining the eyes, ears, peripheral lymph nodes, the limbs, thoracic cavity (including cardiac auscultation) and abdominal cavity

DERMATOLOGICAL EXAMINATION

- check for evidence of ectoparasites
- feel the skin — thickened? (hypothyroidism), atrophic? (hyperadrenocorticism), inflamed? (hypersensitivity disorders), cool? (hypothyroidism)
- examine the lesions
- localized or generalized, symmetrical or asymmetrical?

Primary lesions

- macules: circumscribed area of colour change. Pigmentary disturbances
- papules: solid elevated lesions < 1.0 cm in diameter. Folliculitis, hypersensitivity
- plaques: elevated lesions occupying a large surface area. Hypersensitivity
- nodules: palpable solid, circumscribed, deep. Neoplasia, deep infection
- pustules: look like papules but pus can be expressed. Pyoderma
- vesicles: rarely seen (thin epidermis). Viral disease, autoimmune disease, acute trauma
- epidermal collarette. Rupture of a vesicle or pustule; there is a rim of peeling epidermis surrounding an erosion, which tends to undergo hyperpigmentation as it heals

Secondary lesions

- scales, crusts, scabs, ulcerations and excoriation due to self-trauma
- lichenification (thickened, elephant-like skin). Chronic inflammation
- hyperpigmentation. Chronic inflammation and chronic endocrinopathies
- alopecia. Self-trauma, follicular damage, endocrinopathy
  Having taken a history and made a physical examination and dermatological examination, all data are noted, and lesion distribution recorded on a line diagram.
- in many instances a diagnosis is suggested at this point, and

laboratory and other diagnostic tests may now be performed to confirm the diagnosis
• in other instances, it will be necessary to make a list of differential diagnoses, beginning with the most likely. Subsequent investigations into each disease on the list are then undertaken

GENERAL LABORATORY AND OTHER DIAGNOSTIC TECHNIQUES

Haematology

• eosinophilia may be present in type I hypersensitivity reactions, in feline eosinophilic granuloma and in flea-bite hypersensitivity
• eosinopenia and lymphopenia occur frequently in hyperadrenocorticism
• hypothyroid dogs may exhibit a normocytic, normochromic non-regenerative anaemia, leucopenia, lymphocytosis and thrombocytopenia

Biochemistry

• investigation of liver, kidney, pancreatic and gastrointestinal disorders which may cause secondary skin lesions
• hypercholesterolaemia is a common finding in hypothyroidism, hyperadrenocorticism and diabetes mellitus

Biopsy

• essential for the diagnosis of neoplastic and autoimmune disorders
• useful for some parasitic, fungal and skin conditions
• full-thickness biopsies are necessary and if possible some normal tissue should be included. Biopsy punches are obtainable from Stiefel Laboratories, Slough, United Kingdom
• send full details to the histopathologist, who should be familiar with canine and feline histopathology
• samples are sent to the laboratory in 10% formalin for routine histopathology and in Michel's medium for immunofluorescence (obtainable from the laboratory processing the biopsy)

Techniques for the diagnosis of ectoparasites

• direct observation; use magnifying lens and good lighting
• coat brushings; useful for flea faeces and *Cheyletiella*
• adhesive tape; stick tape to clipped skin, then transfer to glass slide

Skin scrapings

• skin scrapings are an essential part of the investigation of most dermatological cases
• it is the most effective way of confirming canine scabies, demodicosis, feline scabies and cheyletiellosis
• select a site typical of the disease in question, avoiding traumatized areas, squeeze the skin, moisten with cotton wool soaked in mineral oil, and scrape with a scalpel blade
• deep scrapings (resulting in slight capillary ooze) are essential for *Sarcoptes*, *Notoedres* and *Demodex*; shallow scrapings are satisfactory for *Cheyletiella*
• the material collected is transferred on to a glass slide, a coverslip is placed and examination is made using the low power of the microscope. Alternatively, scrapings may be taken with a blade moistened in 5% potassium hydroxide, and clearing under a coverslip obtained with the same solution
• allow adequate time for examination of the slide — some mites, notably *Sarcoptes*, are difficult to find
• concentration and flotation of mites can be performed by gently simmering all the material from scrapings in a test-tube with 10% potassium hydroxide until the debris dissolves. Centrifuge and discard the supernatant, half fill the test-tube with saturated sugar solution; then centrifuge at 1000 rev/min; examine the surface film for mites and/or ova

Techniques for the diagnosis of bacterial infection

• *Staphylococcus intermedius* is considered to be the most important pathogen in pyoderma cases (see p. 8)
• only intact pustules are swabbed; these are prepared with 70% alcohol prior to swabbing; the pustule is opened with a 25-gauge sterile needle and, after sampling, the swab is sent to the laboratory in transport medium

Techniques for the diagnosis of mycotic infection

• the ultraviolet (Wood's) lamp is a useful screening test for *Microsporum canis*. It is important to warm the lamp for a few minutes prior to use, and to perform the examination in a dark room
• affected hairs fluoresce apple-green, although not all affected hairs will exhibit fluorescence
• direct microscopy in 5% potassium hydroxide or mineral oil may detect spores and hyphae
• fungal culture

- culture of the fungus is the most reliable method of diagnosing mycotic infection. The medium used is Sabouraud's dextrose agar, under aerobic conditions
- specific fungal identification is by examination of the colony morphology and the microscopic appearance of the macroconidia in wet preparations. This is usually best undertaken by an experienced mycologist
- dermatophyte test medium (DTM) is Sabouraud's dextrose agar with added phenol red. A change of colour to red appears 3 to 14 days after inoculation in dermatophyte cases as a result of alkaline metabolites produced by the fungus; after 14 days contaminant fungi produce the colour change; this method may be misleading if incorrectly used
- suitable culture material is fluorescent hairs or broken hairs plucked from lesion sites along with scales and crusts
- asymptomatic carrier animals may be detected by the Mackenzie brush technique; the coat is brushed with a toothbrush sterilized in 0.1% chlorhexidine, and the accumulated hair and scale transferred to the culture medium

Other diagnostic tests are discussed under the relevant diseases.

2/Bacterial Skin Disease (Pyoderma)

Pyodermas are important in small-animal practices. They may be defined as cutaneous pyogenic infections: most are secondary.

CUTANEOUS MICROBIOLOGY

- skin micro-organisms are either residents (able to multiply on the skin) or transients (not able to multiply on the skin)
- examples of residents include α-haemolytic streptococci, coagulase-negative micrococci and *Clostridia* spp.
- examples of transients include *Proteus*, *Pseudomonas* and *Corynebacterium*. These organisms are only of clinical significance as secondary invaders
- *Staphylococcus intermedius* is considered to be the most important cutaneous bacterial pathogen, with *S. aureus* and *S. hyicus* being implicated in a few cases

CLASSIFICATION OF PYODERMA

- pyodermas are most conveniently classified according to the depth of infection (Table 2.1)

SURFACE PYODERMA

- characterized by superficial erosion of the outer layers of the stratum corneum

Table 2.1 Pyoderma classification

Surface
Acute moist dermatitis
Skin fold pyoderma

Superficial pyoderma
Impetigo
Superficial folliculitis

Deep pyoderma
Muzzle folliculitis and furunculosis
Nasal pyoderma
Interdigital pyoderma
Pressure point pyoderma
German shepherd dog pyoderma
Pyotraumatic folliculitis
Generalized cellulitis and furunculosis

- although *Staphylococcus intermedius* may be isolated in these cases the role of bacteria is not considered to be so important as in the deeper infections and it is not standard practice to culture and perform sensitivity tests
- investigation of the underlying cause and its treatment will ensure prompt recovery in most cases

Acute moist dermatitis (pyotraumatic dermatitis, hot spots)

- any breed of dog — particularly long-haired
- tends to occur more frequently in hot humid weather
- self-trauma perpetuates the problem (itch—lick—chew cycle)
- lesions develop rapidly — typical sites include the neck, face, tail base and hind legs (Fig. 1)
- possible underlying causes are listed in Table 2.2

Table 2.2 Underlying causes in acute moist dermatitis

Flea-bite hypersensitivity (the most important)
Other ectoparasites
Anal sac infection, impaction
Neurosis
Endoparasites (hypersensitivity)
Otitis externa
Superficial bite wounds
Contact irritants
Atopy
Food hypersensitivity
Musculoskeletal disorders, e.g. arthritis
Poor grooming, dirty unkempt coat
Foreign bodies
Idiopathic

Diagnosis

- history
- physical examination
- consideration of the underlying causes in Table 2.2

Differential diagnosis

- demodicosis
- dermatophyte infection
- neoplasia
- candidiasis
- deep pyoderma

Treatment

- attend to the underlying cause
- clip gently — consider sedation
- bathe with shampoos, e.g. 0.5% hexetidine (Hexocil, Parke-Davis)
- short-term topical or parenteral glucocorticoids with antibacterial agents; 7 to 10 days is usually sufficient

Note that glucocorticoids are contra-indicated in deeper pyodermas

Skin fold pyoderma (intertrigo)

Skin folds are anatomical defects. Friction and poor ventilation in association with a warm humid environment favour bacterial multiplication. This condition is found in various sites.

Lip fold pyoderma

- lower lip
- spaniels particularly
- acute moist dermatitis develops in the fold. The dog may be presented with an owner complaint of halitosis, and bad teeth may be part of the problem, particularly if there is hypersalivation. It is useful to swab with a cotton bud to determine if the fold is the main source of the halitosis

Treatment

- surgical: correction of the fold (cheiloplasty)
- medical: 2.5% benzoyl peroxide shampoo (Oxydex, C-Vet)

Facial fold pyoderma

- brachycephalic breeds, such as the Pekingese and British bulldog are predisposed (Fig. 2)
- the fold may irritate the cornea causing ulceration

Treatment

- medical management may be possible as for lip fold pyoderma
- the most effective treatment is surgical, although the owner may not agree as the appearance of the dog will be changed and the dog no longer conform to the breed standard

Vulvar fold pyoderma

- perivulvar dermatitis

- usually found in bitches that have been spayed before their first oestrus and are obese; any breed
- there is excess licking around the vulva, and there may be a foul odour
- pull the vulva upwards to demonstrate the acute inflammation within the fold (this is easily missed if the examination is cursory) (Fig. 3)

Treatment

- surgical: episoplasty
- medical: reduce weight; shampoos as for lip fold pyoderma

Tail fold pyoderma

- corkscrew tail
- particularly found in the Boston terrier, British bulldog

Treatment

- medical: as for lip fold pyodermas
- surgical: correction of the defect

Body fold pyoderma

- Chinese shar pei predisposed
- obese individuals of any breed

Treatment

- weight reduction
- medical: as for lip fold pyoderma

SUPERFICIAL PYODERMA

These are defined as bacterial infections at the level of the intact hair follicle or the epidermis immediately below the stratum corneum.

Impetigo (juvenile pustular dermatitis, 'puppy pyoderma')

Definition

Subcorneal pyoderma affecting mainly the glabrous skin of the ventral abdomen and axillae.

Clinical features

- young puppies prior to puberty
- pustules, papules and yellow scabs
- relatively benign condition, may be asymptomatic
- non-contagious (unlike human impetigo)
- may be associated with poor husbandry; check for ectoparasites, endoparasites, poor nutrition and unhygienic environment

Treatment

- treat the underlying cause
- antibacterial shampoos, e.g. ethyl lactate (Etiderm, Virbac) 0.5% hexetidine, 2.5% benzoyl peroxide
- 7−10 days of narrow-spectrum antibacterial agents such as erythromycin (only needed if the first two methods do not bring about prompt resolution)
- do not use glucocorticoids either topically or systemically (see under superficial folliculitis)

Superficial folliculitis

Definition

Bacterial infection at the level of and including the intact hair follicle.

Clinical features

- any age but more common in young dogs
- any breed
- variable lesions — pustules with hair protruding, papules, crusts, localized 'moth-eaten' alopecia, and epidermal collarettes (Figs 4−6)
- the variety of lesions may contribute to difficulty in recognition of the problem as folliculitis
- most cases show variable degrees of pruritus, with occasional cases being non-pruritic

Underlying factors

Consider:
- seborrhoea
- trauma
- flea-bite hypersensitivity

- scabies
- demodicosis
- atopy
- food hypersensitivity
- contact hypersensitivity
- endocrine changes at puberty
- hyperadrenocorticism
- hypothyroidism
- dermatophytosis (note that lesions of bacterial folliculitis may be erroneously diagnosed as dermatophytosis)

Diagnosis

- history
- physical examination
- examination of stained smears of pus and/or bacterial culture
- intact pustules, if present, should be carefully swabbed with 70% alcohol, allowed to dry, then pricked with a 25-gauge sterile needle and pus collected for staining with e.g. Diff-Quik (Merz and Dade, Switzerland) and culture
- culture should isolate the most important pathogen *S. intermedius*
- failure to identify or isolate *S. intermedius* should prompt re-sampling and repeat culture
- skin scrapings should always be performed to check for *Demodex*

Treatment

- identify and treat the underlying cause if possible
- antibacterial therapy, topical and parenteral (see deep pyoderma for further detail)
- antibacterial therapy is prescribed for an initial period of 3 weeks, and for an additional 10 days following clinical resolution
- do not use glucocorticoids in any form, even if the dog is pruritic. In uncomplicated cases the pruritus diminishes during effective antibacterial therapy. If the lesions disappear, but pruritus persists, this is a useful indication of a likely underlying pruritic cause, e.g. a hypersensitivity disorder such as atopy. Such diagnostic clues are masked by the use of glucocorticoids, and their use also predisposes to seborrhoea, which together with anti-inflammatory effects usually results in a worsening of the folliculitis

Dermatophilus infection

This is a rare pyoderma in dogs with only a few cases having been reported.

- caused by *Dermatophilus congolensis*, which acts as a secondary invader
- initiating factors are excess moisture (most important), ectoparasites and inflammatory skin conditions

Clinical features

- acute moist dermatitis, seborrhoea, crusting often in association with excess moisture
- exudative purulent dermatitis below raised tufts (paint-brush lesions)

Diagnosis

- direct smear and stain (Giemsa, Wright)
- culture on blood agar
- biopsy

Treatment

- groom
- bathe with povidone iodine (Pevidine)
- systemic antibacterial agents for 7–10 days, e.g. ampicillin, tetracyclines, cephalexin, lincomycin
- avoid excessive moisture

DEEP PYODERMA

Definition

Bacterial infection of the skin beneath the hair follicle involving both dermal and subcuticular tissues.
- less common than superficial pyoderma
- *S. intermedius* is the most important pathogen but other bacteria may have a secondary role
- there is usually less difficulty in recognizing the condition in comparison with the superficial form, due to the presence of pus
- there are always underlying causes
- in localized cases consider foreign bodies such as grass awns, trauma or nail-bed infection
- in generalized cases consider:
  Demodex: always perform skin scrapings
  dermatophyte infection
  hypothyroidism
  hyperadrenocorticism

mismanagement with glucocorticoids
immunodeficiency

Muzzle and chin folliculitis and furunculosis (canine acne) (Fig. 7)

- usually seen in young adult dogs
- more common in Great Danes, boxers, Dobermann pinschers and bulldogs

Clinical features

- lesions consist of papules, pustules, comedones and draining tracts
- these lesions do not usually worry the dog, but invariably the owner is concerned
- spontaneous regression is common at puberty, with a few cases persisting for life

Diagnosis

- history
- physical examination
- perform skin scrapings since *Demodex* is occasionally involved
- smear and stain pus, with e.g. Diff-Quik
- culture and antibacterial sensitivity is not normally necessary, since systemic antibacterial agents are not routinely used

Treatment

- topical and occasionally systemic antibacterial agents (see p. 20)

Nasal pyoderma

- mainly dolichocephalic breeds, relatively uncommon
- possibly starts with local trauma or rooting, although the cause is poorly understood, and the role of bacteria is uncertain
- sudden onset, painful, erythematous swollen lesion on the bridge of the nose (Figs 8 and 9)

Diagnosis

- history
- physical examination
- bacterial culture

Differential diagnosis

Consider:
- demodicosis
- dermatophytosis
- nasal solar dermatitis
- discoid lupus erythematosus
- systemic lupus erythematosus
- pemphigus foliaceus
- pemphigus erythematosus
- zinc-responsive dermatosis

Treatment

- antibacterial agents for at least 3 weeks, some cases requiring 5 to 6 weeks (see p. 20)
- sedation and/or an Elizabethan collar in the initial stages
- lack of response is most likely due to one of the diseases listed above being present, or that an underlying factor exists; most of these are poorly understood at present

Interdigital pyoderma

- short-coated breeds such as the Great Dane, English bulldog, dachshund and Weimaraner are predisposed

Clinical features

- the feet may be swollen, painful and discharge pus
- licking may induce alopecia
- paronychia and pyonychia may occur simultaneously
- in chronic cases nodules, ulceration, fistulae and furunculosis
- regional lymph nodes may be enlarged

Diagnosis

- history
- physical examination
- staining of smears
- bacterial and fungal culture
- skin scrapings
- radiology of the feet to check for bony change

Underlying factors

Consider:
- foreign body (one foot usually involved)

- trauma (stones, gravel, stubble)
- contact irritants (e.g. fertilizers, sand, tar, chemicals)
- contact hypersensitivity
- food hypersensitivity
- drug eruption
- atopy
- autoimmune disease
- dermatophyte infection
- *Demodex canis*
- *Neotrombicula autumnalis*
- *Ancylostoma*
- *Uncinaria*
- psychogenic factors
- hypothyroidism
- hyperadrenocorticism
- immunodeficiency
- zinc-responsive dermatosis
- idiopathy

Treatment

- identify the underlying cause and treat if possible
- surgical drainage
- bathe the feet in saline
- systemic antibacterial agents — for 20 days beyond clinical cure
- autogenous vaccines may be tried in resistant cases in conjunction with the above
- some authorities have used immune stimulators such as levamisole at a dose of 2.2 mg/kg three times weekly. This drug is not licensed for use in the dog and side-effects may occur

Pressure point pyoderma (callus pyoderma)

- usually seen in large dogs such as the Great Dane, St Bernard, any age or sex
- affects the elbows, hocks and sometimes the sternum
- the skin in these areas becomes thickened, and repeated trauma may lead to deep pyoderma (Fig. 10)

Underlying factors

Consider:
- obesity
- lying on hard surfaces
- hypothyroidism
- immunodeficiency — difficult to prove

Treatment

- antibacterial therapy (see p. 20)
- reduce weight
- provide soft bedding
- ablation (high risk of breakdown)
- check thyroid function if the above measures are not successful

German shepherd dog pyoderma

- almost exclusively seen in German shepherd dogs
- middle-aged

Clinical features

- lesions (papules, pustules leading to furunculosis), hyper-pigmentation and alopecia are typically seen on the dorsum, gluteal region, ventral abdomen and thighs
- advanced cases may become generalized, with the head and front feet spared, and there may be a peripheral lymphadenopathy
- affected dogs are usually otherwise in good health

Diagnosis

- history
- physical examination
- bacterial culture
- skin scrapings and fungal culture to rule out fungi and ectoparasites

Treatment

- long-term antibacterial therapy (see p. 20)
- prognosis is poor

Pyotraumatic folliculitis

- more commonly young dogs
- golden retrievers and St Bernards may be predisposed

Clinical features

- mimics acute moist dermatitis
- no response to cleansing and glucocorticoid therapy

Diagnosis

- biopsy — deep, suppurating necrotizing folliculitis

Treatment

- as for deep pyoderma (see p. 20)

Generalized deep folliculitis, furunculosis and cellulitis

- the most severe type of deep pyoderma

Underlying factors

Consider:
- generalized debility
- demodicosis
- dermatophyte infection
- hypothyroidism
- misuse of glucocorticoids

Clinical features

- lesions consist of pustules, crusts, pus-discharging fistulae and alopecia
- these lesions may occur anywhere but are especially pronounced on the trunk and ventral abdomen) (Fig. 11)

Diagnosis

- history
- physical examination
- bacterial culture
- biopsy
- *S. intermedius* is considered to be the most important pathogen, but *Escherichia coli, Pseudomonas* and *Proteus* commonly act as secondary invaders

Treatment

- antibacterial therapy against *S. intermedius* (see p. 20)
- whirlpool bathing in e.g. povidone iodine (Pevidine)

ANTIBACTERIAL THERAPY IN THE MANAGEMENT OF SUPERFICIAL AND DEEP PYODERMA

- assess the depth of infection before beginning therapy
- type, duration and frequency of treatment depend on the above
- some mild cases may be managed with topical therapy alone
- suitable shampoos include hexetidine (Hexocil, Parke-Davis), benzoyl peroxide (Oxydex, C-Vet), ethyl lactate (Etiderm, Virbac) and surgical scrubs such as povidone iodine
- in more severe cases use topical therapy as an adjunct to treatment with systemic antibacterial agents
- systemic antibacterial agents may be employed empirically or be based on bacterial culture and sensitivity testing. Wherever possible, and always in deep pyodermas, sensitivity testing is recommended
- suitable antibacterial agents include erythromycin, lincomycin (Lincocin, Upjohn), clavulanic acid-potentiated amoxycillin (Synulox, Beecham Animal Health) and trimethoprim-potentiated sulphonamides (Tribrissen, Coopers Pitman-Moore)
- cost should be taken into consideration due to the lengthy treatment required
- if *S. intermedius* is not isolated, then reculture is advised, since it is the main pathogen
- if several organisms are isolated with varying antibacterial resistances, choose one of the above that is effective against *S. intermedius*, since elimination of this organism will frequently bring about remission in these cases

Pitfalls in antibacterial therapy

Inadequate dose

- this is usually in large dogs, due to an understandable tendency of the veterinary surgeon to worry about the cost
- weigh the dog and prescribe the recommended dose
- in deep pyodermas the antibacterial agents may be used at twice the recommended dose

Changing the antibacterial agent too soon

- in superficial pyodermas it will usually be a week or two before the lesions begin to clear; thus changing treatment before a 2-week period is not justified, and usually 3 weeks is allowed before making any therapeutic decisions

- at the end of the 3 weeks look for a reduction in pruritus, fewer lesions or resolution of lesions. If there is an improvement continue with the drug

Stopping the treatment too soon

- as a general rule it is advisable to continue antibacterial treatment for 10 days beyond apparent clinical cure in superficial pyoderma cases and for 3 weeks in severe deep pyoderma
- if the treatment is stopped just as the lesions clear, there is usually a relapse
- explain this to the owner at the outset and stress the importance of keeping appointments for rechecks

PYODERMA OF CATS

Feline pyoderma

- the cat does not commonly suffer from bacterial skin disease, except for infections following bites
- bacteria isolated from infected wounds reflect the normal oral flora; *Pasteurella multocida*, β-haemolytic streptococci, *Fusiformis* spp. *Pasteurella* is the most important of these
- cat bite sepsis is most commonly seen in adult males (Fig. 12)

Treatment

- surgery, drainage of abscesses
- systemic antibacterial agents; 5–7 days
- if poor healing, suspect feline leukaemia or immunodeficiency virus
- castration: reduces the incidence by 80%

OTHER LESS COMMON FELINE PYODERMAS

Impetigo

- occasionally seen in young kittens
- pustular dermatitis develops on the back of the neck initially and may spread elsewhere
- cultures reveal *Pasteurella multocida* and/or β-haemolytic streptococci
- infection possibly transferred from the mouth of the queen

Treatment

- gentle cleaning
- 7−10 days of systemic antibacterial agents

Folliculitis

- rare
- papules and pustules associated with hair shafts
- may see moist dermatitis, erosions, crusting, ulceration
- often seen on the chin (secondary to feline acne?) and sometimes spreading to involve the face and body (presenting as a miliary dermatitis)

Diagnosis

- history
- physical examination
- biopsy
- skin scrapings and bacterial culture to rule out demodicosis or dermatophyte infection

Treatment

- gentle cleaning
- systemic antibacterial agents

Feline acne

- seen occasionally in cats of any age or sex (therefore differing from canine acne, which is predominantly confined to adolescence)
- possibly associated with inadequate cleaning of the chin in some cats
- comedones, pustules and papules on the chin and occasionally the lips; oedema of the chin may be seen

Treatment

- gentle daily washing of the chin with warm soapy water (may also be done prophylactically)
- systemic antibacterial agents
- no treatment necessary in mild cases

Feline leprosy

- a rare granulomatous nodular infection of the cat skin

- probably caused by *Mycobacterium lepraemurium* (the rat leprosy bacillus)

Clinical features

- lesions usually on the head and limbs (suggesting infection from rat bites)
- single or multiple nodules
- may ulcerate and drain, non-healing
- the cat is not systemically ill

Diagnosis

- history
- physical examination
- biopsy (acid-fast bacilli in Ziehl–Nielsen stain)

Differential diagnosis

- tuberculosis — extremely rare in countries where the bovine form has been eradicated
- neoplasia
- foreign-body reaction

Treatment

- surgical excision where feasible
- if surgery is impracticable some authorities have used the anti-leprosy drug diaminodiphenylsulphone (dapsone, Ayerst) at a dose of 50 mg/kg b.i.d. Results have been variable, and there is a risk of haemolytic anaemia. This drug is not licensed for use in cats

MISCELLANEOUS UNCOMMON PYODERMAS OF DOGS AND CATS

Cutaneous tuberculosis

- very rare in the UK and in other countries where tuberculosis has been eradicated
- Most infections caused by *Mycobacterium bovis* and *M. tuberculosis* (rarely *M. avium*)

Clinical features

- single or multiple nodules which may discharge a thick yellow pus

- affected animals may be unwell (weight loss, anorexia, lymphadenopathy and intermittent pyrexia)

Diagnosis

- history
- physical examination
- biopsy
- culture (6−8 weeks)
- BCG test (dogs only)

Treatment

- euthanasia is advisable due to the public health risk

Bacterial pseudomycetoma

- rare condition of dogs and cats usually initiated by bites or local trauma
- organisms incriminated include coagulase-positive Staphylococci, *Pseudomonas* spp., *Proteus* spp., *Streptococcus* spp. and *Actinobacillus* spp.

Clinical features

- single or multiple nodules with draining fistulae
- exudate may contain fine white granules

Treatment

- surgical excision with post-surgical antibacterial therapy

Opportunist mycobacterial granuloma

- dogs and cats
- rare condition caused by soil-living bacteria, e.g. *Mycobacterium fortuitum* and *M. chelonei*

Clinical features

- chronic soft-tissue abscessation with ulceration and draining fistulae
- lesions occur on the groin, abdomen and thorax (less commonly on the head)

Diagnosis

- stain exudate with acid-fast stains
- culture
- biopsy

Treatment

- wide surgical excision with postoperative antibacterial cover

Actinobacillosis

- rare disease of dogs and cats caused by *Actinobacillus lignierisi*
- infection usually follows a bite since the above organism is a commensal in the mouth of many animals

Clinical features

- thick-walled abscesses in the skin which discharge pus containing yellow granules.

Diagnosis

- culture
- staining of smears
- biopsy

Treatment

- surgical removal of the lesion
- also suggested is sodium iodide (0.2 ml/kg of 20% solution orally twice daily) and antibacterial therapy (sulphonamides, tetracyclines, chloramphenicol and streptomycin)

Actinomycosis

- many species, including dogs and cats
- rare disease caused by *Actinomyces* spp.
- infection from trauma and local wounds

Clinical features

- signs may take months to years to develop
- cutaneous abscesses or granulomas with osteomyelitis in disseminated lesions

- fistulae may develop which discharge a foul-smelling exudate containing 'sulphur granules'

Diagnosis

- culture
- staining of smears
- biopsy

Treatment

- high-dose long-term antibacterial therapy with penicillin, sulphonamides or trimethoprim-potentiated sulphonamide

Nocardiosis

- rare disease causing systemic infections or purulent infections of body cavities, bone, central nervous system and skin
- organisms incriminated include *Nocardia asteroides*, *N. braziliensis* and *N. caviae*, which are usually found in the soil

Clinical features

- ulcerated nodules, most commonly on the limbs
- these nodules discharge a tomato soup-like exudate
- usually an associated lymphadenopathy
- body cavity involvement leads to pyothorax and/or purulent ascites

Diagnosis

- culture
- smear
- biopsy

Treatment

- drainage of lesions
- long-term antibacterial agents
- the antibacterial agent of choice is clindamycin (Antirobe, Upjohn) and with this agent the prognosis is reasonable
- other antibacterial agents are less effective

Borreliosis (lyme disease)

- recently recognized in dogs

- rare
- caused by the tick-transmitted spirochaete *Borrelia burgdorferi*
- may manifest as pyotraumatic dermatitis at the site of tick-bites

Diagnosis

- history
- physical examination
- biopsy
- serology

Treatment

- oral tetracyclines are effective

3/Parasitic Skin Disease

FLEAS

- the most common cause of skin disease in the dog and cat
- the most frequently found species affecting both dogs and cats is the cat flea *Ctenocephalides felis*
- other species also encountered on dogs and cats include:
  Ctenocephalides canis (dog)
  Leptosylla segnis (rat)
  Echidnophaga gallinacea (chicken)
  Archeopsyllus erinacei (hedgehog)
  Spilopsyllus cuniculi (rabbit)
  Pulex irritans (human)

Life cycle

The life cycle is 3 weeks to 2 years.
- the female lays eggs (3−18) in the environment or on the host and may live 1−2 years, laying up to 500 eggs in that time
- incubation varies according to temperature and relative humidity; under optimum conditions the eggs hatch in 2−4 days
- larvae ingest faecal pellets and develop over three stages to pupae and finally adults; under unfavourable conditions the life cycle can take up to 2 years
- unfed adults can survive 3 months away from the host
- it is now considered by most authorities that cutaneous reactions to fleas are the result of the development of hypersensitivity to flea saliva

Flea-bite hypersensitivity (flea-allergic dermatitis)

Clinical features

DOGS
- very common
- hypersensitivity develops to haptens in the saliva and both immediate and delayed hypersensitivity responses occur
- wheals, erythema and papules develop at the site of flea-bites; these can be anywhere on the body, but particularly on the dorsum, tail head, hind legs and ventral abdomen (Fig. 13)
- self-trauma from licking and scratching causes acute moist dermatitis in the early stages, and seborrhoea, lichenification and alopecia in chronic cases

- the condition tends to be seasonal in the UK (not in warm climates)

CATS
- flea-bite hypersensitivity in the cat usually presents as miliary dermatitis
- occasional cases mimic 'endocrine alopecia' (Fig. 14), or have isolated patches of acute moist dermatitis or eosinophilic plaques

Diagnosis

- physical examination
- identification of fleas or flea excrement; the latter may be differentiated from dirt particles by placing them on wet blotting-paper; a reddish tinge diffuses out from the flea excrement
- lesions in typical sites — the dorsum, tail head, backs of thighs, ventral abdomen
- intradermal testing using flea extract. These are available in the United States[*] and Holland[†]
- response to a flea eradication programme. In the United Kingdom, except during the very warm, humid times of the year, usually late August, it is possible to eradicate fleas from the environment; in warm climates this is very difficult and not useful as a diagnostic test

Differential diagnosis

DOGS
- folliculitis
- other ectoparasites
- food hypersensitivity
- atopy. Many dogs that are hypersensitive to flea-bites are also atopic
- drug eruption
- endoparasite hypersensitivity

CATS
- as for miliary dermatitis (see pp. 166–167)
- feline symmetric alopecia

Treatment

OWNER
EDUCATION
- essential; time must be spent on this
- explain the life cycle of the flea

---

[*] Flea extract 1:1000, Greer Laboratories, Lenoir, North Carolina.
[†] HAL Allergen Laboratories, Haarlem, Holland.

• in flea hypersensitivity it is useful to use as an analogy the allergic reactions which many people have to midge or mosquito bites. It is usually obvious to the owner that considerable pruritus and self-trauma can be initiated by only a few fleas

FLEA CONTROL

• must be comprehensive
• treat the animal and all those in contact with insecticides, such as in shampoos, sprays or powders
• treat the environment with a combination of permethrin and methoprene (Acclaim plus, Ceva Ltd). Methoprene is a juvenile insect hormone analogue, which prevents the flea larvae pupating
• in persistent cases it is useful to call in a professional pest control company
• prevent reinfestation of the environment by repeating all the above measures regularly during the summer months
• flea collars are of limited use in a flea control programme
• the particular flea control programme used depends on each individual case and is best worked out between the veterinary surgeon and the animal owner. Experience, tact, common sense and time are the most important requisites in formulating a control programme

GLUCOCORTICOIDS

• these should be used only for a short term in the early stages of treatment, or if for any reason flea control is impractical
• prednisolone is the drug of choice and is best administered on an alternate-day basis. It is preferable to educate the owner that a slight degree of pruritus in the animal is more acceptable than the development of iatrogenic hyperadrenocorticism due to the mis-management of glucocorticoids. Most such cases seen by the author have received long-acting repositol injectable glucocorticoids. These are not necessary in the management of hypersensitivity disorders
• the treatment of flea-bite hypersensitivity in the cat is discussed under miliary dermatitis (see pp. 166–167)

LICE

• host-specific
• survive only a few days if separated from the host
• the life cycle is entirely on the host: 14–21 days; eggs hatch to nymphs, two or three moults to adult
• lice are either biting (suborder Mallophaga) or sucking (suborder Anoplura)
• Canine species include:
    Trichodectes canis (biting)

Linognathus setosus (sucking)
Heterodoxus spiniger (biting), warm climates
- Feline species: *Felicola subrostratus* (biting)

Clinical features

- infestation with lice is called pediculosis
- clinical features are variable
- asymptomatic carrier
- seborrhoea sicca
- variable pruritus
- if pruritus is severe, secondary alopecia and excoriation
- lesions similar to flea-bite hypersensitivity in the dog
- lesions similar to miliary dermatitis in the cat
- mouse-like odour to the coat
- anaemia in heavy infestations (*Linognathus setosus*)

Underlying factors

- poor sanitation
- matted ungroomed coat
- old age and debility
- overcrowding

Diagnosis

- identify the lice by physical examination
- examine with a magnifying lens as lice are easily overlooked

Differential diagnosis

- seborrhoea
- flea-bite hypersensitivity
- *Cheyletiella* spp.
- *Sarcoptes scabiei*
- other ectoparasites
- hypersensitivity disorders

Treatment

- lice are susceptible to most insecticides, and insecticidal shampoos are therefore effective in both dogs and cats
- repeat treatments after 10 days
- treat the environment

• attend to underlying diseases and improve the animal's living conditions
• clean grooming implements

TICKS

• two classes: hard (ixodid) and soft (argasid)
• occur in all species, all breeds and either sex
• many species affect both dogs and cats, depending on geography and climate
• most problems are caused by hard ticks; the only soft tick of importance is the spinous ear tick, *Otobius megnini*, found in warm climates
• In the United Kingdom common ticks are *Ixodes ricinus* (the 'castor bean' tick), *Ixodes canisuga* and *Ixodes hexagonus* (the 'hedgehog tick' — but also found on dogs and cats)

Life cycle

This has a species variability of 2 months to 3 years. A typical ixodid life cycle is as follows:
• eggs laid on the ground
• hatch in 2–7 weeks
• larvae feed on the host (3–12 days), drop off, rest (6–90 days) and moult
• nymphs feed on the host (3–12 days), drop off, rest (17–100 days) and moult
• adults may live up to 3 years; females are capable of laying between 2000 and 8000 eggs in their lifetimes

Clinical features

There are various possibilities.
• asymptomatic
• owner notices 'cyst'
• skin irritation due to bites
• hypersensitivity reactions
• anaemia if infestation is heavy
• paralysis (certain species in Australia and the United States)
• vectors for bacterial, rickettsial, viral and protozoal disease

Diagnosis

• physical examination

Treatment

• Manual removal; apply an ether swab first, or spray with an insecticidal agent. Care must be taken to remove the entire tick or a foreign-body granuloma will develop
• insecticidal shampoos and sprays
• treat the environment if possible, with insecticidal sprays
• prophylaxis by regular spraying of the environment, and the use of insecticides as sprays, powders, shampoos or collars on the animal
• if a foreign-body granuloma develops at the site of attachment, remove surgically

MITE INFESTATION

Cheyletiella (cheyletiellosis, walking dandruff) (Fig. 15)

• canine species: *Cheyletiella yasguri*
• feline species: *Cheyletiella blakei*
• three other species have been described in rabbits and hares
• cross-infection between species is possible

Life cycle

This takes place entirely on the host and lasts about 5 weeks.
• adult lays eggs, hatch into larvae, nymph 1, nymph 2 and adult
• adults live for about 14 days in the keratin layer of the epidermis; they do not burrow
• survival off the host is not usually more than 2 days except in cold conditions when survival of up to 10 days is possible

Clinical features

DOGS   • common
• most cases occur in puppies, especially from pet shops, occasionally breeding establishments; often detected at physical examination prior to vaccination
• excessive scale is the principal sign (usually very noticeable) (Fig. 16)
• pruritus is variable but often absent in young puppies

CATS   • less common than in dogs; long-haired breeds may be predisposed
• may have excessive scale similar to puppies
• sometimes develop a miliary dermatitis-type response (Fig. 17)

- may be asymptomatic
- in both cats and dogs human lesions are very commonly found in contact sites, such as the abdomen, when the cat or dog has been sitting on the owner's lap. There may be a history of treatment by the family doctor for a non-specific rash, or the doctor may request veterinary examination of the pet

Diagnosis

- laboratory confirmation is essential, especially if human lesions have developed; the family doctor and the kennel owner/pet shop owner must be informed. Any doubts expressed by third parties are quickly dispelled by an invitation to view the mite under the microscope

Techniques of diagnosis include:
- transparent adhesive tape pressed on to the surface of scaly skin and then transferred to a glass slide
- superficial skin scraping, using mineral oil to ensure that the material adheres to the scalpel blade; usually many mites and eggs are found by this method
- coat brushings: the debris is collected, cleared with 10% potassium hydroxide, centrifuged and the deposit added to saturated sugar solution. After a few hours the surface of the supernatant is examined for mites
- hair pluckings: hair from scaly areas is plucked and placed between two glass slides and eggs searched for. *Cheyletiella* eggs are cocooned and often numerous. This method is particularly valuable in cats, since in this species adult mites may be difficult to find (Fig. 18)
- direct examination of coat brushings
- in severe cases the mites may be observed in motion (walking dandruff); usually large numbers of mites and an efficient magnifying lens are necessary

Differential diagnosis

- *Otodectes cynotis*
- *Sarcoptes scabiei*
- *Notoedres cati*
- *Dermanyssus gallinae*
- *Neotrombicula autumnalis*
- lice
- flea-bite hypersensitivity
- *Pelodera* spp.
- primary idiopathic seborrhoea

Treatment

- antiparasitic shampoos such as 1% gamma benzene hexachloride (Quellada, Stafford-Miller) or 1% selenium sulphide (Seleen, Ceva Ltd); three shampoos at weekly intervals are necessary
- treat all in-contact animals
- treat the environment with insecticidal powders or sprays, then vacuum clean
- if the above measures are carried out efficiently, human lesions will clear spontaneously within 3 weeks

Notoedres cati (feline scabies, notoedric mange)

- disease of cats (but also reported in dogs, foxes and rabbits) and caused by *Notoedres cati*
- life cycle similar to *Sarcoptes scabiei*
- extremely rare in the United Kingdom

Clinical features

- lesions start on the ears and spread to the face, eyelids and neck
- later lesions may appear on the feet and perineum, and become more generalized if untreated
- lesions consist of crusts, scabs, partial alopecia and in chronic cases lichenification
- there is intense pruritus

Differential diagnosis

- *Otodectes cynotis* infestation
- dermatophyte infection
- pyoderma secondary to fight wounds
- *Cheyletiella* spp.
- lice
- food hypersensitivity
- pemphigus complex
- systemic lupus erythematosus
- atopy

Treatment

- parasiticidal shampoo such as 1% selenium sulphide (Seleen, Ceva Ltd) or gamma benzene hexachloride (Quellada, Stafford-Miller)
- glucocorticoids and antibacterial therapy

- insecticidal powders and sprays for the environment (mites can survive 3–4 days off the host)
- treat all in-contact cats

Sarcoptes scabiei (canine scabies, sarcoptic mange) (Fig. 19)

- an intensely pruritic parasitic skin condition of dogs caused by *Sarcoptes scabiei* var. *canis*
- primarily a mite infesting dogs, but may also affect cats, foxes and man

Life cycle

The life cycle is 3–4 weeks.
- adults copulate on the surface of the skin
- female adult burrows into the skin and lays 3 to 4 eggs per day
- larvae hatch and return to the surface to develop into nymphs
- nymphs develop into adults
- adults live for 3–4 weeks and can only survive off the host for 2–3 days

Clinical features

- scabies is highly contagious, mostly by direct contact, but grooming instruments and kennels may harbour mites
- the condition is highly pruritic, anti-inflammatory doses of glucocorticoids frequently failing to control pruritus
- rubbing the pinna of the ear between the thumb and forefinger frequently elicits a scratch reflex
- typical lesions are papules and crusts, especially on the pinnae, elbows, brisket and limbs
- lesions become generalized if not treated, and hyperpigmentation with lichenification and lymphadenopathy may occur (Fig. 20)
- human lesions in contact sites are common

Diagnosis

- history
- physical examination
- skin scrapings: clip the hair and look for small papules. Multiple scrapings should be taken from these lesions. Excoriated lesions are poor scraping sites. Spend adequate time looking for mites — at least 30 minutes — and if unsuccessful perform concentration and flotation of the scrapings, using 10% potassium hydroxide to digest keratin and saturated sugar solution to float the mites

- even with multiple skin scrapings and prolonged searching for the mites, positive identification may not be made
- if the mite is not found, but scabies is still strongly suspected a therapeutic trial should be undertaken as described below. If the dog responds to treatment and remains cured, this allied to clinical signs makes a retrospective diagnosis of scabies acceptable
- only perform a therapeutic trial after a very careful search for the mite in multiple skin scrapings

Differential diagnosis

- hypersensitivity disorders (atopy, food hypersensitivity, contact hypersensitivity)
- scabies is frequently misdiagnosed as one of the above diseases. An increasing degree of pruritus which is poorly controlled by anti-inflammatory doses of glucocorticoids should alert the clinician to the possibility of infestation with *Sarcoptes scabiei*. Before undertaking expensive and time-consuming hypersensitivity investigations it is wise to treat for scabies
- most owners will accept the logic of the above measures with good communication
- *Cheyletiella*
- *Otodectes*
- lice
- other causes of seborrhoea
- other underlying causes of pyoderma
- *Pelodera* spp.

Treatment

- clip long-haired dogs; this is essential to allow penetration of antiparasitic shampoos
- the treatment of choice in the UK is 1% gamma benzene hexachloride shampoo (Quellada, Stafford-Miller) The shampoo is left on for 5 minutes prior to rinsing off, and repeated weekly for 3 weeks
- short-term glucocorticoids parenterally; 7 days is adequate — longer than this will mask successful therapy
- spray the kennels with insecticide
- examine the dog after 3 weeks' treatment. If there has been no reduction in pruritus, check that the owner is treating the dog as instructed; there may have been inadequate instruction in the shampooing process or the owner may not be able to cope with it. Consider shampooing the dog in the hospital with trained staff. Rarely it may be necessary to change to another parasiticide such as

bromocyclen (Alugan, Hoechst)
• treat all in-contact dogs
• human lesions will normally clear spontaneously with effective treatment of the dog within a few weeks, since the canine mite cannot complete its life cycle on human skin
• other treatments reported to be effective in the treatment of canine scabies but not licensed in the UK include Amitraz and Ivermectin

Demodex canis (demodicosis, demodectic mange, follicular mange, red mange) (Fig. 21)

• demodicosis is a disease of dogs caused by *Demodex canis*
• this mite is a normal inhabitant of canine skin, but is found in much larger numbers in diseased dogs
• the mite is an obligate parasite inhabiting the hair follicles and occasionally the sebaceous glands

Life cycle

• this is incompletely understood. There are, however, four stages: eggs, six-legged larvae, eight-legged nymphs and eight-legged adults
• mites are transferred from the bitch to the nursing neonates in the first 2−3 days of life only. Thereafter the disease is non-contagious
• the mites cannot survive away from the host; the entire life cycle is therefore spent in the skin

Clinical features

• any breed, age or sex; more common in pure-bred dogs, and also in short-haired breeds
• some long-haired breeds are susceptible, such as the Old English sheepdog, Afghan hound, German shepherd dog, collie and West Highland white terrier
• three forms of the disease are recognized: localized (squamous) demodicosis, generalized demodicosis and demodectic pododermatitis

LOCALIZED DEMODICOSIS
• most cases in pups 3−6 months old (Fig. 22)
• lesions typically develop on the head and forelegs, less commonly on the trunk
• patchy alopecia with mild erythema and scaling; later hyperpigmentation

• the majority of cases undergo spontaneous regression without treatment, with approximately 10% of cases developing the generalized form of the condition

GENERALIZED
DEMODICOSIS

This can be further subdivided into:
• juvenile-onset
• adult-onset
• demodectic pododermatitis

Juvenile-onset demodicosis

• this is the term used to describe cases beginning before the age of 2 years
• most common form of generalized demodicosis
• numerous lesions, appear rapidly on the head, legs and trunk; alopecic patches, scaling, erythema or lichenification, depending on the length of time affected before examination
• some cases, especially in the initial stages, do not have secondary pyoderma and are termed squamous (Fig. 23)
• secondary pyoderma, however, is a common complication and this is the most severe form of demodicosis
• such cases have been shown to have severe T-lymphocyte suppression
• the exact cause of this T-cell suppression is yet to be determined. Scott and others (1976) suggested that affected dogs may have an inherited specific immunoincompetence for *Demodex canis* which allows the mite to multiply in large numbers, and that the mites produce a humoral substance which further depresses the immune system
• Barta and others (1983) noted the immune depression to be present only when there was a secondary pyoderma and therefore suggested that the pyoderma was the cause of the immune depression
• when there is secondary pyoderma, *Staphylococcus intermedius* is usually isolated, and in more severe cases *Pseudomonas* and *Proteus* may also be isolated

Adult-onset demodicosis

• rare
• signs first seen in dogs that are older than 2 years
• may be associated with debilitating, immunosuppressive diseases or the injudicious use of glucocorticoids in high doses. In many cases it is extremely difficult to establish an underlying cause, and such cases tend to recur following treatment and need lifelong therapy
• warn the owner of this fact and also of the possibility of underlying serious systemic disease or neoplasia
• the lesions and their distribution are essentially the same as for juvenile-onset demodicosis (Fig. 24)

Demodectic
pododermatitis
• foot lesions are common in generalized demodicosis, but some cases present with foot lesions as the only clinical sign
• there is thickening of the skin with hyperpigmentation, and secondary pyoderma is common
• there may be pain and oedema
• some cases may result from a generalized case which has not completely responded to treatment

Diagnosis

Skin scrapings are essential.
• squeeze affected skin before scraping
• deep scrapings are necessary
• all deep pyodermas must have skin scrapings performed since *Demodex* is an important underlying cause
• similarly all pododermatoses should be checked for *Demodex*
• in generalized cases the mite is present in large numbers and therefore easy to find
• in chronic pododermatitis *Demodex* is sometimes detected by biopsy, as the extreme thickening of the skin may impede the diagnosis by skin scraping
• hair pluckings using epilation forceps are frequently successful in detecting mites

Differential diagnosis

• generalized pyoderma
• dermatophyte infection
• canine acne
• seborrhoea
• pemphigus complex
• dermatomyositis

Treatment

LOCALIZED
DEMODICOSIS
• most cases resolve spontaneously with or without treatment (provided that glucocorticoids are *not* used)
• daily applications of a 3% solution of rotenone
(Head to Tail Veterinary Demodectic Mange Dressing, Coopers Pitman-Moore)
• warn the owner that cases may appear to deteriorate initially as diseased hairs fall out

GENERALIZED
DEMODICOSIS
• many 'cures' reported in the literature; most of dubious value
• some juvenile-onset cases will recover spontaneously with or without treatment

There are two recommended treatments in the UK: Amitraz (Derasect Demodectic Mange Wash, Beecham Animal Health) and Rotenone (Head to Tail Veterinary Demodectic Mange Dressing, Coopers Pitman-Moore).

Amitraz (Figs 25 and 26)

- clip hair
- bathe with e.g. 2.5% benzoyl peroxide to remove crusts and flush follicles
- Amitraz solution (5% w/v) is diluted 1:100 in water and the entire body soaked. Use gloves and perform the procedure in a well-ventilated room
- dry — do not rinse off
- repeat weekly (consider performing the procedure in the hospital if there is any doubt about the owner's ability to comply)
- antibacterial cover is essential in those cases with secondary pyoderma; these agents are used as in the discussion under pyoderma (p. 20)
- continue treatment until the dog is clinically normal and multiple skin scrapings are negative on two occasions two weeks apart (usually 10−12 weeks)
- some cases relapse following cessation of treatment; these cases may require prolonged (occasionally lifelong) treatment, but they are the exception and the success rate of the above treatment is good, given owner compliance

Rotenone

- clip the dog
- the solution is diluted with 3 equal parts of spirit immediately before use
- apply to one-third of the body daily, using a different site for each application in rotation
- use antibacterial agents if there is secondary pyoderma
- 1% selenium sulphide shampoo weekly is a useful adjunct to treatment. This preparation removes excess scale and debris and is also acaricidal
- the above is continued until the dog is clinically normal and multiple skin scrapings are negative on two occasions with an interval of two weeks between them
- this method is extremely effective but requires much more effort from the owner and most unsuccessful cases are due to lack of compliance

Glucocorticoids are contra-indicated in the management of demodicosis

- dogs are likely to be already immunosuppressed and glucocorticoids will make matters worse. In addition secondary pyoderma will be encouraged
- do not breed from animals that have recovered from any form of demodicosis, or that have produced pups with the disease

- such animals are best neutered since the condition tends to be inherited, and relapse of apparently cured animals may occur at oestrus

Demodex cati (**feline demodicosis**)

- rare
- two species have been described in the cat — *Demodex cati* and an unnamed species which is shorter and blunter (Figs 27 and 28)
- localized form more common than generalized

Clinical features

LOCALIZED DEMODICOSIS
- patchy alopecia, erythema and hyperpigmentation; head, peri-ocular area and neck
- variable pruritus
- some cases present as a ceruminous otitis

GENERALIZED DEMODICOSIS
- alopecia, scaling and hyperpigmentation; head, neck and legs
- may mimic feline symmetric alopecia
- may mimic feline scabies, particularly if the unnamed species is involved

Diagnosis

- skin scrapings
- consider possible underlying disease, e.g. feline leukaemia virus infection, feline immunodeficiency virus, diabetes mellitus, auto-immune disorders. Some cases have been seen after prolonged megestrol acetate therapy

Differential diagnosis

- feline symmetric alopecia
- feline psychogenic alopecia
- dermatophytosis
- atopy
- food hypersensitivity
- feline scabies
- flea-bite hypersensitivity

Treatment

- clip the coat if long-haired
- weekly shampoos with 1% selenium sulphide

Otodectes cynotis (ear mites) (Fig. 29)

- found in both the dog and the cat
- mites are just visible to the naked eye (white dots) and occur mainly in the ear canal, but may be found on the neck, gluteal region and tail

Life cycle

This lasts 3 weeks.
- eggs hatch into six-legged larvae, develop into eight-legged protonymphs and then deutonymphs
- deutonymphs are approached by adult males; copulation occurs if the deutonymph develops into a female

Clinical features

- otitis externa with thick, waxy discharge
- less frequently crusting, papular lesions on the neck, gluteal region and head, which may mimic flea-bite or hypersensitivity
- such cases may be due to hypersensitivity to the mite (Fig. 30)
- human lesions have been reported
- mites may survive off the host for months

Treatment

- aural miticidal preparations, such as GAC (Dales Pharmaceuticals Ltd), Otoryl (May and Baker Ltd) or Auroid (Willows Francis)
- acaricidal powder/spray — entire body, especially the tail in cats, since the tail is often in close contact with the ears when the animal is sleeping
- treat the environment with acaricidal sprays
- glucocorticoids may be necessary if hypersensitivity develops (7–10 days is sufficient provided that ectoparasitic control is thorough)

Neotrombicula autumnalis (harvest mites, chiggers) (Fig. 31)

- common, especially chalky soils
- N. autumnalis is the commonest species in the UK
- other species (USA) include Eutrombicula alfreddugesi

Life cycle

This takes between 50 and 70 days:

• adult lives in organic decaying material: eggs hatch to six-legged larvae which are parasitic. The larvae attack dogs and cats and many other species including man. The natural hosts are thought to be small rodents such as field mice
• the larvae drop to the ground and develop into nymphs and then adults
• adult females may live for 1 year
• the parasitic larvae only emerge in late summer and autumn

Clinical features

DOGS   • pododermatitis, severe if hypersensitivity develops (Fig. 32)

CATS   • may be non-pruritic papules and crusts on the limbs
• more usually intense pruritus on contact sites (feet, ventral abdomen and ears)

Diagnosis

• seasonal, late summer and autumn only
• mites can be seen (bright orange dots) with the naked eye, between the toes, on the legs and around the pinna of the ear and in Henry's pocket of the ear (especially in cats)
• may also be detected in skin scrapings from lesion sites
• mites remain on the host for 3–15 days

Treatment

• antiparasitic washes
• glucocorticoids parenterally (5–7 days only)
• avoid grassland, woods during the season

Dermanyssus gallinae (red mite of poultry)

• natural host is poultry
• also attacks wild and caged birds, dogs, cats and man

Life cycle

This lasts between 7 days and 5 months, depending on feeding.
• adult lives in nests, cages; female lays up to 7 eggs, which hatch into non-feeding six-legged nymphs
• after a few days eight-legged protonymphs, then deutonymphs, and finally adults emerge
• most problems in dogs and cats are associated with access to

chicken houses, very occasionally with birds nesting in the house

Clinical features

- any age or sex, cats and dogs
- pruritus with papules, crusts and erythema on the limbs and back particularly

Diagnosis

- history of exposure to poultry or wild birds
- skin scrapings and identification of the mite

Treatment

- antiparasitic washes
- environmental acaricidal sprays
- glucocorticoids if the pruritus is severe

Lynxacarus radovsky (cat fur mite)

- found in Australia, Hawaii, Florida
- does not usually cause symptoms
- in heavy infestations with attachment to the outer half of the hair shafts, the coat is given a 'salt-and-pepper' appearance and loses its lustre

Diagnosis

- coat brushings, skin scrapings, impressions with transparent adhesive tape
- identify the mite

Treatment

- acaricidal shampoos weekly for 3–4 weeks
- treat all in-contact animals
- treat the environment

FLIES (DIPTERA)

Stomoxys calcitrans (stable fly)

- the stable fly occasionally bites dogs housed indoors
- lesions tend to be on the face and ears

Treatment

- house dogs indoors during the day
- insecticidal sprays and creams may help to deter the flies from biting
- topical glucocorticoid creams

Myiasis (fly strike)

- more commonly affects old dogs and cats
- two families of flies cause myiasis; blowflies (calliphorids) and flesh-flies (sarcophagids)

Life cycle

This lasts usually 1−4 weeks.

CALLIPHORIDS
- eggs are laid on skin lesions (see underlying factors)
- larvae hatch into pupae which develop into adults
- adults may live for about 1 month

SARCOPHAGIDS
- deposit larvae, not eggs

Clinical features

- favoured sites for fly strike are the anus, genitalia and occasionally the nose
- large numbers of larvae (maggots) are found at these sites and there is usually tissue necrosis

Underlying factors

- urinary or faecal incontinence
- other skin diseases, e.g. pyoderma
- constant lacrimation or salivation
- general debility, lack of grooming, associated with old age or any serious neglected illness

Treatment

- clip lesion site
- clean the wounds
- extract the larvae
- use antibacterial agents
- shampoo the rest of the coat with an insecticidal agent

- attend to underlying factors

Cuterebra maculata (cuterebriasis)

- dogs and cats
- warm climates (not United Kingdom)
- normal host is the rabbit and other rodents

Life cycle

- adults (bee-like) lay eggs near burrows or nests of rodents
- dogs and cats pick up eggs in contaminated areas
- larvae penetrate the skin or are ingested, and undergo aberrant migration
- those larvae in the skin are typically found around the head and neck

Clinical features

- swellings of about 1 cm in diameter which develop an air hole

Diagnosis

- physical examination

Treatment

- incise air hole and carefully extract larva
- take care not to crush the larva — risk of anaphylaxis

BEES, WASPS (HYMENOPTERA)

- not parasites, but included here
- dogs and cats, particularly puppies and kittens
- local oedema, pain and erythema at the site of the sting
- rarely anaphylactic shock

Treatment

- remove sting
- glucocorticoids by injection
- antihistamines
- adrenaline and intravenous glucocorticoids for anaphylactic shock
- usually signs disappear within 24 hours

HELMINTH PARASITES

Uncinaria stenocephala, Ancylostoma caninum (hookworm dermatitis)

- dogs of any age, sex or breed
- particularly seen in groups of kennelled sporting dogs on grass or earth runs

Life cycle

- eggs are deposited on the ground; moisture is important for development
- cutaneous lesions are caused by percutaneous entry of third-stage larvae, but most larvae penetrating by this route do not mature
- *U. stenocephala* is the main species seen in the UK
- this species does not suck blood

Clinical features

- dermatitis in contact sites — sternum, ventral abdomen, lateral and posterior aspects of carpal, metacarpal regions and pads
- there may be erythema, oedema and pain in the pads, which often have a spongy texture in the early stages (Fig. 33)
- in chronic cases the pads become hyperkeratotic, ulcerated and cracked; paronychia and nail deformities may also be features

Diagnosis

- history
- physical examination
- biopsy; there is a disruption of the epidermis with tortuous tracks in the dermis infiltrated by neutrophils and eosinophils; there may also be dermal oedema and perivascular cuffing
- presence of hookworm eggs in the faeces, in association with clinical signs

Treatment

- anthelminthics such as nitroscanate (Lopatol, Ciba-Geigy)
- avoidance of contaminated runs
- salt or sodium borate may be used to kill the parasite on the ground

Pelodera (Rhabditis) strongyloides (Pelodera dermatitis)

- dogs, any age, sex or breed
- not reported in dogs in the UK (but may occur)
- caused by the larvae of the free-living nematode *Pelodera strongyloides*

Life cycle

- direct: adults live in decaying organic matter
- females may be either parthenogenetic or oviparous
- larvae invade the skin of the animal

Clinical features

- pruritus at ventral contact sites
- papules, crusts, intense erythema
- secondary infection is common

Diagnosis

- history
- skin scrapings — larvae
- biopsy

Differential diagnosis

- hookworm dermatitis
- dirofilariasis
- dermatophyte infection
- primary irritant dermatitis
- contact hypersensitivity
- demodicosis
- scabies

Underlying factors

- insanitary conditions
- dampness
- presence of warm organic debris

Treatment

- insecticidal shampoos
- clean the bedding

- spray the environment with insecticide
- glucocorticoids parenterally for a few days initially

Dirofilaria immitis (**dirofilariasis, heartworm**)

- warm countries — not seen in the UK
- dogs of any breed or sex
- larvae of *Dirofilaria immitis* are occasionally found in subcutaneous tissue

Clinical features

- nodules
- pruritic ulcerative dermatitis
- focal alopecia
- severe pruritus resembling scabies
- poor or no response to antibacterial and glucocorticoid therapy

Diagnosis

- demonstrate microfilariae in blood samples
- biopsy: microfilarial segments in blood vessels

Treatment

- thiacetarsamide and dithiazanine
- thiacetarsamide and Ivermectin

Dracuncula insignis (**dracunculiasis**)

- found in North America
- dogs of any age, sex or breed

Life cycle

- dogs acquire infection by ingesting crustaceans which act as intermediate hosts
- larvae develop in 8—12 months into adults, which inhabit the subcutaneous tissue of the abdominal wall and the limbs

Clinical features

- discrete single nodules
- these have a drain hole and the nodule contains the worm (25—50 cm in length)

Diagnosis

- history
- physical examination
- smears of exudate from the drain hole contain larvae
- biopsy

Treatment

- surgical excision
- metronizadole or diethylcarbamazine have been suggested

PROTOZOA

Leishmania canis (leishmaniasis)

- occurs in dogs from endemic areas (Mediterranean countries, Middle East, some parts of Africa and Central America)
- transmitted by sandflies
- *Leishmania* tends to concentrate in the reticuloendothelial system and the skin

Clinical features

- lesions in the skin are pruritic nodules, with a dry exfoliative dermatitis
- the nodules may ulcerate, and tend to occur at biting sites such as the head or ears
- there may be anaemia, intermittent pyrexia, generalized lymphadenopathy, weight loss, hepatosplenomegaly and lethargy

Diagnosis

- history
- physical examination
- biopsy: skin lesions, lymph nodes, bone marrow
- the parasite is found both intracellularly and extracellularly and is best seen with Giemsa stain
- indirect immunofluorescent antibody test and other serological tests (Longstaffe and Guy 1985)

Treatment

- meglumine antimonate (Glucantime)
- sodium stibogluconate (Pentostam)

- metronidazole (Flagyl) and ketoconazole (Nizoral, Janssen) have also been tried
- relapse is frequent and cure may be difficult to achieve
- it may be necessary to consider euthanasia in view of the difficulty of treatment and the possibility of human infection

RICKETTSIA

Rickettsia rickettsii (Rocky Mountain spotted fever)

- dogs
- tick transmission
- USA only

Clinical features

- fever
- anorexia
- skin lesions: erythema, petechiation, especially ventral skin, pinnae (in males epididymitis, scrotal ulceration)

Diagnosis

- history
- physical examination
- haematology: anaemia, leucopenia, thrombocytopenia
- skin biopsy: necrotizing vasculitis

Treatment

- tetracyclines for 3 weeks
- nursing and supportive therapy

4/Fungal Skin Disease

SUPERFICIAL MYCOSES

These are fungal infections that involve the skin, hair and nails.

Dermatophytosis (ringworm)

• dermatophytosis is the term used for infection with species of *Microsporum*, *Trichophyton* or *Epidermophyton*. Dermatomycosis is the term used for infection with non-dermatophytes
• almost all cases of dermatophytosis in the dog or cat are caused by fungi of the genera *Microsporum* or *Trichophyton*
• the fungi attack the keratin of the hair only in the anagen phase of the growth cycle

Clinical features

DOGS
• dermatophytosis in the dog is rare in the United Kingdom
• prevalence (Wright 1989) in the UK is:
   M. canis 65%
   T. mentagrophytes (mouse or vole) 23%
   T. mentagrophytes var. *erinacei* (hedgehogs) 5.2%
   M. persicolor (mouse or vole) 4%
   T. verrucosum, *T. terrestre*, *M. gypseum* (soil) 1.6%
• infection is by direct contact with an infected animal or contaminated material from the environment
• in healthy animals dermatophytosis is a self-limiting disease; young animals which lack acquired immunity or any animal with compromised immunity (particularly cell-mediated) are susceptible
• lesions are variable and include circular patchy alopecia (Fig. 34), erythematous plaques, folliculitis, scales and crusts. The lesions may be localized or diffuse, and occasionally involve large parts of the body — especially with *T. mentagrophytes* (Fig. 35). Infection may involve the nails (onychomycosis), which break off and subsequently grow back deformed. Other lesions resemble a histiocytoma, with severe inflammation and secondary infection (kerion Fig. 36). Secondary infection may lead to hair loss and scarring

CATS
• 98% of infections are with *M. canis* (Fig. 37), the remainder being due to *T. mentagrophytes*
• very common

53

- any age, sex or breed, but particularly young animals
- lesions in the owner are very common
- lesions in the cat are variable and include circular 'cigarette-ash' patches of alopecia, miliary dermatitis-like lesions and crusts, or may be asymptomatic

Diagnosis

- Wood's lamp examination: a useful screening test. Of the important pathogenic fungi, fluorescence is only seen in certain strains of *M. canis*
- the fluorescence is due to a tryptophan metabolite produced by the fungus
- it is important to warm the lamp up for 5 minutes to achieve the correct wavelength, and to examine the animal in a darkened room
- affected hairs fluoresce bright green. False fluorescence may be caused by certain ointments, soaps and powders containing, for example, oxytetracycline
- a negative test does not rule out dermatophytosis
- potassium hydroxide preparation: suspect infected hairs are mounted in 10% KOH or KOH-DMSO, and examined for fungal hyphae or arthrospores, which are seen as small, spherical, refractile bodies in chains or in a mosaic sheath around the hair. Staining with lactophenol cotton blue or blue-black ink may facilitate identification of the arthrospores
- fungal culture: ideally fluorescent hairs or hairs with broken roots should be selected at the periphery of the lesion. In addition skin scrapings can be made from the centre of the lesion. Where there are no lesions material can be collected with a sterile toothbrush and transferred to the culture medium (Mackenzie brush technique)
- the medium employed for culture is Sabouraud's dextrose agar. Dermatophytes are identified by their colony morphology, and by characteristic macro-aleurospores, which are usually produced after approximately three weeks' incubation at room temperature. Their identification is a specialized task and the details are not discussed in this text. In the hands of a competent veterinary mycologist, fungal culture is the most reliable means of diagnosing dermatophytosis in the dog and cat
- dermatophyte test medium (DTM) is based on Sabouraud's dextrose agar with phenol red added as an indicator. Pathogenic dermatophytes metabolize protein, producing alkaline metabolites which induce a red coloration in the medium. This change in colour occurs normally at between 3 and 7 days (occasionally up to 14 days). Saprophytic fungi metabolize carbohydrate first, and produce alkaline metabolites much later. Thus any colour change will occur after 14 days

- DTM cultures should be examined daily and considered negative if there is no colour change before 14 days. They are best used in conjunction with plain Sabouraud's dextrose agar, since used alone they do not allow identification of the dermatophyte species
- biopsy: staining with periodic acid Schiff (PAS) will often reveal septate fungal hyphae and spores, either on hairs or within the hair follicle or stratum corneum

Differential diagnosis

- superficial pyoderma
- demodicosis
- seborrhoea
- contact dermatitis
- histiocytoma
- acral lick dermatitis
- mast cell tumour
- mycosis fungoides
- pemphigus complex

Treatment

- many cases will undergo spontaneous resolution
- griseofulvin (Grisovin, Coopers Pitman-Moore) is the drug of choice for severe, widespread or chronic cases
- the dose suggested is 20–100 mg/kg daily, with severe cases requiring the higher dose
- the drug is given with a high-fat meal or with vegetable oil to facilitate absorption
- do not administer griseofulvin to pregnant animals as it is teratogenic
- clipping the coat, especially in long-haired cats, is essential (burn the clippings)
- topical treatment with 0.2% enilconazole (Imaverol, Jannsen) in dogs or the sodium salt of benzuldazic acid (Defungit, Hoechst) in the cat is a useful adjunct to therapy
- ketoconazole (Nizoral, Jannsen) is an alternative to griseofulvin, and has been used at a dose of 15 mg/kg. It does not have a product licence in the dog and cat, and side-effects (hepatotoxicity, vomiting and pruritus) have been reported

Control of dermatophyte infection in kennels and catteries

- this is an arduous and time-consuming task
- good communication with, and co-operation from, the owner is most important

- all in-contact animals should be screened with the Wood's lamp and by culture, using the Mackenzie brush technique
- infected animals are treated with griseofulvin until negative on two consecutive cultural examinations one month apart
- negative in-contacts are treated topically as above for two weeks
- burn as much contaminated material in the premises as possible
- effective disinfectants include formalin, 0.2% enilconazole, sodium hypochlorite and steam
- paint woodwork to seal in infection
- spores may remain viable for a year or more; thus environmental treatment should be as thorough as realistically possible

Candidiasis

- infection of the mucous membranes and skin caused by *Candida albicans*
- very rare
- mainly dogs

Clinical features

- ulceration (white-grey plaques) of the mucous lining of the cheeks and ventral surface of the tongue; there may be a foul-smelling discharge
- vaginal discharge
- otitis externa
- acute moist dermatitis near mucocutaneous junctions
- paronychia

Diagnosis

- direct smear: stain with lactophenol cotton blue
- culture: Sabouraud's dextrose agar
- biopsy: the organism may be seen in the stratum corneum after routine staining with haematoxylin and eosin (H and E) or with special stains such as periodic acid Schiff (PAS)

Differential diagnosis

- stomatitis
- acute moist dermatitis
- causes of otitis externa
- fold pyoderma
- pemphigus vulgaris, bullous pemphigoid
- dermatophytosis

Underlying factors

- prolonged administration of antibacterial agents
- immunosuppression or deficiency
- concurrent debilitating diseases
- persistent moisture

Treatment

- correct underlying cause
- topical, for example miconazole (Conaderm, C-Vet) or enilconazole (Imaverol, Janssen)
- systemic, for example ketoconazole (Nizoral) orally (possible side-effects are vomiting, hepatotoxicity and pruritus) or amphotericin B (danger of nephrotoxicity; see systemic mycoses, pp. 62)
- neither of the above drugs is licensed for use in the dog

Malassezia pachydermatitis (Pityrosporum canis)

- *M. pachydermatitis*, a yeast, is a normal commensal of the ears which occasionally is associated with otitis externa
- rarely a more generalized dermatosis may occur and Scott and Muller (1989) have reported on a series of young West Highland white terriers which presented with a severe pruritic seborrhoeic disorder from which pure growth of the yeast was obtained on skin culture
- it is suggested that these dogs have a genetically determined epidermal dysplasia predisposing to *M. pachydermatitis*

Diagnosis

- aural swabs or skin scrapings followed by staining (Diff-quik, methylene blue) or culture in Sabouraud's dextrose agar
- biopsy may demonstrate the yeast in the epidermis

Treatment

- many aural preparations contain antifungal agents
- it is more important to identify and treat the underlying cause of the otitis
- failure to treat the underlying cause will inevitably mean recurrence of pathogenic numbers of yeast organisms following apparently successful symptomatic treatment
- oral ketoconazole (Nizoral, Janssen) was used successfully by Scott and Muller (1989) in the generalized seborrhoeic form at a

dose of 10 mg/kg. Cessation of therapy was invariably followed by relapse.

SUBCUTANEOUS MYCOSES

- infection by fungi of viable skin, often traumatically induced
- very rare in the UK
- examples include eumycotic mycetoma, phaeohyphomycosis, pythiosis, protothecosis and sporotrichosis
- identification of these fungi should be undertaken only by an experienced veterinary mycologist

Eumycotic mycetoma

- rare in dogs and cats
- trauma-induced, may involve the skin, subcutaneous tissue, fascia and bone
- causal fungi include *Allescheria boydii* and *Curvularia geniculata*
- causal actinomycetes include *Actinomyces* and *Nocardia*

Clinical features

- frequently there is a triad of swelling, draining fistulae and granules
- usually localized lesion, typically on a foot
- may be painful and swollen

Diagnosis

- culture on plain Sabouraud's agar
- histopathology: demonstration of fungal elements with specialized stains such as PAS

Differential diagnosis

- abscesses
- foreign body reactions
- neoplasms

Treatment

- radical surgical excision
- there is no effective medical therapy

Phaeohyphomycosis

- mainly cats, a few cases have been reported in dogs

- rare
- causal fungi in cats include *Drechslera spicifera*, *Phialophora verrucosa*, *Moniella suaveloens* and *Exophiala jeanselmii*
- causal fungi in dogs include *D. spicifera*, *Phialemonium obovatum* and *Pseudomichrodochium suttonii*

Clinical features

- early lesions are painless subcutaneous nodules
- later, fistulation occurs with a purulent exudate
- ulceration may occur
- lesions tend to form on the distal extremities and trunk

Diagnosis

- culture on plain Sabouraud's agar

Differential diagnosis

- chronic abscessation
- foreign-body reaction
- feline leprosy
- eumycotic mycetoma

Treatment

- surgical excision
- amphotericin B or ketoconazole may be tried

Pythiosis (Phycomycosis)

- rare
- dogs
- warm climates only, e.g. south-eastern United States
- usually seen in dogs that have access to stagnant water
- caused by fungi of the genus *Pythium* (often pathogens of aquatic plants)

Clinical features

- ulcerated nodules on the limbs, posterior dorsum and tail or face
- may develop fistulae with a serosanguinous or purulent exudate

Diagnosis

- culture from material collected surgically from the centre of lesions

Differential diagnosis

- other fungal infections
- deep pyoderma
- demodicosis
- acral pruritic granuloma
- neoplasms

Treatment

- radical surgical excision of the lesion (amputation of affected portion of a limb may be necessary)
- antifungal medical therapy is ineffective

Protothecosis

- rare
- dogs and cats
- causal agents are achlorophyllous algae related to the green algae *Chlorella* spp.
- *Prototheca wickerhamii* is the only species to have been recovered from dogs and cats
- there has been a report of this condition in the UK in a 10-year-old greyhound (Macartney *et al.* 1988)

Clinical features

- small nodules which may ulcerate and discharge a thick exudate
- these nodules may occur on the limbs, nose, chest and head
- may spread to the regional lymph nodes

Diagnosis

- culture on plain Sabouraud's agar
- biopsy and stain with PAS

Differential diagnosis

- deep pyoderma
- fungal infections
- neoplasms
- atypical mycobacterial infections
- systemic mycoses with skin manifestations

Treatment

- surgical removal of nodules in early stages

- ketoconazole may be tried but the condition is usually refractory to treatment

Sporotrichosis

- rare
- dogs and cats
- warm climates only
- public health risk
- causal fungus is *Sporothrix schenkii*
- there are three clinical syndromes:
  cutaneolymphatic: nodules on the skin of the extremities, infection spreading to the regional lymph nodes; the nodules rupture with a red-brown discharge
  cutaneous: circumscribed, alopecic, plaque-like non-painful lesions
  disseminated: invasion of many tissues

Diagnosis

- culture on Sabouraud's dextrose agar
- biopsy

Differential diagnosis

- chronic ulcerative conditions
- granulomas
- other mycoses
- feline leprosy
- deep pyoderma

Treatment

- the cutaneous and cutaneolymphatic forms respond well to inorganic iodide therapy

DOGS 0.2 mg/kg of a 20% solution of sodium iodide is given orally b.i.d. for four weeks beyond clinical remission; at this dose (40 mg/kg) improvement should be noticed within a week

CATS A lower dose (20 mg/kg) is recommended, since cats are more susceptible to iodinism
- toxic signs in the dog include vomiting, depression and seborrhoea sicca
- in the cat there may be vomiting, depression, anorexia and cardiac depression

SYSTEMIC MYCOSES

• Mainly caused by inhalation of conidia, with subsequent pulmonary infection and dissemination to other organs
• causal fungi are saprophytes living in soil or organic matter
• non-contagious
• examples are blastomycosis, coccidioidomycosis, histoplasmosis and cryptococcosis. These diseases are usually only seen in parts of North America
• cryptococcosis has been reported in the UK

Cryptococcosis

• dogs and cats
• causal agent is the yeast-like fungus *Cryptococcus neoformans*, a soil saprophyte, especially in soil contaminated with pigeon droppings
• infection is opportunistic, occurring in animals debilitated or immunosuppressed (e.g. feline leukaemia virus or feline immunodeficiency virus infection, neoplastic conditions or during treatment with anti-cancer drugs)
• rare
• infection acquired via respiratory system with dissemination to the rest of the body

Clinical signs

• cutaneous lesions consist of nodules or papules in the dermis or subcutis
• nodules may ulcerate and develop into crusting lesions or abscesses
• the lesions are most commonly found on the head
• there may be regional lymphadenopathy

Diagnosis

• staining of exudate with methylene blue
• biopsy
• culture on Sabouraud's dextrose agar

Treatment

• surgical excision if feasible (early lesions), together with ketoconazole at a dosage of 10 mg/kg b.i.d. for several months, may be successful but the outlook is guarded

5/Viral Skin Disease

Cowpox

- uncommon
- mainly rural cats
- infection may be from a rodent reservoir — not all affected cats have contact with cattle

Clinical features

- papules, ulcers and particularly scabs develop at the site of cuts or bites, usually the head, neck or limbs
- these lesions may become generalized to involve the entire body and oral mucous membranes, particularly if there is concurrent debilitating disease, or immunosuppressing viral infections such as feline leukaemia or feline immunodeficiency virus infection, or if glucocorticoids have been administered
- affected cats may suffer from a transient dullness, but are not usually unwell; in a minority of cases there is dyspnoea, pyrexia, anorexia and depression
- pruritus is commonly noted

Diagnosis

- history
- physical examination
- virus isolation in tissue culture; send scabs and swabs in viral transport medium to the virology laboratory. Biopsy; eosinophilic intracytoplasmic inclusion bodies within keratinocytes
- serological investigation, e.g. complement fixation, haemagglutination inhibition or neutralization tests. May be of limited value in immunosuppressed cats and acutely ill cats

Differential diagnosis

- bacterial folliculitis
- ectoparasites
- miliary dermatitis
- dermatophyte infection

Treatment

- supportive nursing
- antibacterial agents to prevent secondary infection
- glucocorticoids are contra-indicated since they may cause the infection to become generalized
- resolution may take up to 2 months

Feline leukaemia virus (FeLV) infection

Feline leukaemia virus, due to immunosuppressive activity, may initiate or exacerbate a number of skin diseases; the most important of these are:
- paronychia, particularly chronic and resistant cases
- recurrent or chronic abscessation or cellulitis. There is frequently a history of response to antibacterial agents with rapid relapse when therapy ceases
- seborrhoea
- poor wound healing

Diagnosis

- history
- physical examination
- bacterial and fungal culture, skin scrapings (rule-outs)
- positive virus tests

Treatment

- advise owner of the poor prognosis
- euthanasia

Feline immunodeficiency virus (FIV)

- FIV is associated with a multiplicity of clinical signs including gingivitis, stomatitis, neurological signs and chronic skin disease, particularly pyoderma

Diagnosis

- positive virus tests

Treatment

- euthanasia if severe disease
- supportive therapy in milder cases

Feline herpes virus infection

- uncommon
- superficial ulceration of the skin and oral cavity
- there is a variable course; most cases recover, a few die
- diagnosis is by isolation of the virus from lesions

Treatment

- supportive nursing
- antibacterial cover

Feline calicivirus infection

- rarely associated with cutaneous signs
- reported cases had ulceration of the footpads, swollen painful feet and ulceration of the tongue, palate and lips

Canine distemper

- in some cases of distemper there is a hyperkeratosis of the nose and footpads (Fig. 38)
- in these dogs the planum nasale becomes hard and rough, and there may be fissures; the footpads are thickened, dry and cracked, and walking may be painful
- recovery from distemper often leads to an improvement or resolution of the clinical signs

Diagnosis

- history
- physical examination
- rule out other diseases

Differential diagnosis

- ichthyosis
- nasodigital hyperkeratosis
- pemphigus foliaceus
- discoid lupus erythematosus
- systemic lupus erythematosus
- zinc-responsive dermatosis

Treatment

- trim excessive keratin

- bathing to hydrate the keratin
- apply petroleum jelly after bathing
- topical antibacterial ointments

Papovavirus

Causes cutaneous and mucosal papillomas in the dog (see p. 126)

Feline sarcoma virus

Causes cutaneous fibrosarcoma in young cats (see p. 133)

Contagious ecthyma (orf)

- primarily a sheep and goat disease caused by a paravaccinia virus
- a few cases have been reported in dogs fed on sheep carcases
- acute moist dermatitis, crusts and ulceration occur round the mouth and head

Diagnosis

- history
- physical examination
- virus isolation

Treatment

- supportive nursing
- recovery may take up to 4 weeks

6/Endocrine Skin Disease

GENERAL POINTS

- many hormones affect the skin and adnexa, for example, thyroid hormones, glucocorticoids, growth hormone, oestrogens and androgens
- most commonly the earliest cutaneous sign of a cutaneous disorder is a non-pruritic bilaterally symmetrical alopecia
- pruritus, when it occurs, is usually due to a secondary pyoderma or seborrhoea
- control of hormone levels is by the hypothalamus and pituitary gland as a result of feedback mechanisms from the target endocrine gland
- important hormones secreted by the anterior lobe of the pituitary gland (adenohypophysis) are:
  adrenocorticotrophic hormone (ACTH)
  thyroid-stimulating hormone (TSH)
  growth hormone (GH)
  prolactin
  follicle-stimulating hormone (FSH)
  luteinizing hormone (LH)
  melanocyte-stimulating hormone (MSH)

HYPOTHYROIDISM

- the commonest endocrine disorder of the dog
- the acquired naturally occurring condition has not been documented in the cat although the extremely rare congenital form has been described
- the metabolically active thyroid hormones are L-thyroxine (T4) and L-3,5,3-triiodothyronine (T3)

Aetiology

PRIMARY
- congenital agenesis (rare)
- non-functional thyroid tumour (rare)
- lymphocytic thyroiditis; the most important cause (approximately 90%), an autoimmune disorder which results in thyroid destruction
- idiopathic thyroid necrosis and atrophy may represent the end stage of lymphocytic thyroiditis

SECONDARY
- Less common than primary causes (less than 5%)
- TSH deficiency leading to inadequate stimulation of the thyroid gland with subsequent reduction in the production of thyroid hormone
- congenital hypopituitarism (usually in association with GH deficiency)
- pituitary neoplasia (may present with other signs, e.g. diabetes insipidus)

TERTIARY
- thyrotropin-releasing hormone (TRH) deficiency results in deficiency of TSH and reduction in thyroid hormone production
- due to hypothalamic lesions — extremely rare
- other equally rare causes of hypothyroidism include:
  iodine deficiency
  defects in thyroid hormone synthesis (dyshormonogenesis)
  antithyroid hormone antibodies
  abnormality in plasma iodine binding or T_4 to T_3 conversion

Clinical features

- any age but most likely between 6 and 10 years of age; onset tends to be earlier in the giant breeds
- any sex
- certain breeds are reported to be predisposed, such as the bulldog, boxer, Great Dane, Dobermann, poodle, Scottish terrier, dachshund, Irish wolfhound, Newfoundland, Afghan hound, golden retriever and miniature schnauzer

History

Careful history-taking is particularly important in suspect hypothyroidism cases. The disease has been called 'the great impersonator'. There may be:
- a gradual onset in lethargy and depression
- thermophilia — heat-seeking and unwillingness to go out in cold weather
- gradual onset of poor exercise tolerance
- obesity — this is variable, some dogs may be of normal weight or thin
- slow regrowth of hair after clipping

Physical signs

These are extremely variable and any one or more of the following may be present:

CUTANEOUS
- cool skin
- bilaterally symmetrical alopecia
- hyperpigmentation, thickening of the skin and scaling seborrhoea
- secondary pyoderma (probably associated with depressed immune system function)
- pruritus is absent unless there is a secondary pyoderma or seborrhoea
- dull coat, hairs easily epilated
- puffy skin (myxoedema)
- easy bruising
- hypertrichosis
- comedones

GASTRO-INTESTINAL
- occasional vomiting, diarrhoea or constipation
- none of these are common

CARDIOVASCULAR
- there may be bradycardia
- weak apex beat, low voltage on ECG recordings
- cardiac arrhythmias

REPRODUCTIVE
- irregular oestrus cycles or anoestrus
- decreased libido
- testicular atrophy
- gynaecomastia and galactorrhoea (rarely)

OCULAR
- blepharoptosis
- corneal lipidosis
- keratoconjunctivitis sicca and corneal ulceration
- retinopathy

NEUROMUSCULAR
- facial and laryngeal paralysis
- myopathy, e.g. of the temporal and masseter muscles

Diagnosis

- history, physical examination, laboratory investigation

Laboratory findings

NON-SPECIFIC
- normocytic, normochromic, non-regenerative anaemia is seen in approximately 25% of cases
- hypercholesterolaemia occurs in approximately 33% of cases (sample the fasting dog only)
- serum creatinine phosphokinase (CPK) is often elevated
- skin biopsy: may see hyperkeratosis, epidermal atrophy, melanosis,

follicular atrophy and increased dermal thickening. These signs are consistent with an endocrinopathy and not specific for hypothyroidism

• circulating thyroid hormone concentrations. Total T4 (TT4) is measured by radioimmunoassay. The normal TT4 range is 13−52 nmol/l
• extremely low levels of TT4 (< 7 nmol/l) together with compatible clinical signs support the diagnosis of hypothyroidism
• There is considerable overlap between TT4 levels in some normal dogs and in dogs with hyperthyroidism. Some drugs, such as phenobarbitone, diphenylhydrantoin and glucocorticoids, depress thyroid hormone levels. Chronic systemic diseases also depress thyroid hormone levels ('euthyroid sick syndrome'). To overcome these problems further diagnostic tests are required
• TSH response test
    blood is collected into a plain tube
    5 IU of bovine TSH are given intravenously
    a second blood sample is collected 4 hours later
    allow to clot, centrifuge and separate serum
    send both samples to a laboratory accustomed to canine testing
        and request measurement of TT4
Interpretation: Normal dogs will at least double the basal TT4 and fall within or exceed the normal post-TSH TT4 range for the laboratory. Hypothyroid dogs may show an increase in TT4 levels but they will not reach the normal post-TSH TT4 level.

Further refinements to both the non-dynamic and dynamic function tests have been suggested recently (Larsson 1988). Using the equation:

$$k = 0.7 \times \text{free thyroxine (FT4) concentration (nmol/l)} - \text{cholesterol concentration (mmol/l)}$$

hypothyroid dogs are diagnosed by having a k value less than −4, whereas euthyroid dogs have a k value of greater than +1.

The TSH test accuracy was improved by using the equation:

$$k = 0.7 \times \text{basal TT4 concentration (nmol/l)} + \text{increase in TT4 concentration after TSH (nmol/l)}$$

Hypothyroid dogs have a k value of less than 15, whereas euthyroid dogs have a k value of greater than 30.
• thyroid biopsy. Not commonly employed in practice, but will distinguish between euthyroidism, primary and secondary hypothyroidism, lymphocytic thyroiditis and idiopathic necrosis and atrophy

Treatment

- the drug of choice is thyroxine sodium (Eltroxin, Glaxo) at a dose of 10–20 μg/kg b.i.d. Start therapy at the lower dose and only proceed to the higher dose if the dog fails to respond after a few months. Caution should be exercised with dogs suffering from cardiovascular disease by introducing the drug gradually
- overdosage is difficult to achieve, and side-effects are therefore rare; if encountered they are principally panting, anxiety, restlessness, tachycardia, polyphagia, polyuria and diarrhoea
- the half-life of T4 is 24 hours and peak plasma levels occur 4–12 hours after administration
- most authorities suggest the use of T3 in those cases that fail to improve on T4. However, Thoday (1990) states that he has never seen a dog with hypothyroidism respond to T3 having failed to respond to T4 and the author agrees with this statement
- it is important to ensure that an adequate dose is given and for a sufficient length of time. If lethargy was a notable symptom, this is often the first sign to disappear, dogs regaining vitality within a few weeks. Other signs, particularly alopecia, may take months to improve. It is recommended that a minimum of three months of treatment is given prior to making clinical assessments. Treatment, once established as beneficial to the dog, is for *life*

HYPERADRENOCORTICISM

Also called Cushing's syndrome, this is principally a problem of the dog. It is extremely rare in the cat.

Causes

- pituitary-dependent — 80% of dogs. Excessive ACTH secretion results in adrenocortical hyperplasia and excess secretion of cortisol. According to Peterson *et al*. (1982), most of these cases (80%) are due to microadenomas. Only a few dogs have large pituitary tumours and these are slow-growing and not usually malignant. Very occasionally, neurological signs will develop in these cases
- some pituitary-dependent cases not associated with tumours may be due to a failure of the negative feedback response by cortisol
- the remaining 15–20% of naturally occurring cases are caused by unilateral or bilateral adrenal tumours
- a further significant cause of hyperadrenocorticism is glucocorticoid abuse ('iatrogenic hyperadrenocorticism'). The commonest cause of this is the excessive use of injectable repositol gluco-

corticoids. It is difficult to estimate the number of iatrogenic cases of hyperadrenocorticism occurring, but it is likely that they are of equal importance to naturally occurring cases

Clinical features

- any breed, but particularly toy and miniature poodles, boxers, dachshunds and terrier breeds
- any sex, but females more likely to develop adrenal tumours
- any age, but more common in middle to old age

Clinical signs

GENERAL

Can be any one of the following:
- polyuria, probably due to glucocorticoids inhibiting the secretion or action of antidiuretic hormone
- polydipsia, secondary to the polyuria
- polyphagia, direct effect of glucocorticoids; a few animals, however, are anorexic
- skeletal muscle atrophy, particularly the temporal muscles, shoulders, thighs and pelvic muscles
- weakness, due to the muscle atrophy
- hepatomegaly: in conjunction with abdominal muscle atrophy this often leads to a pendulous abdomen (Fig. 40)
- anoestrus, clitoral enlargement
- testicular atrophy
- panting in approximately one-third of cases; severe dyspnoea may develop as a consequence of heart failure or pulmonary thrombosis
- neurological signs (associated with macroadenomas of the pituitary gland or neoplasia of the adrenal cortex with metastasis)
- lameness, pathological fractures (osteoporosis, osteomalacia)

CUTANEOUS

- bilaterally symmetrical non-pruritic alopecia (not the head or the feet)
- hyperpigmentation
- very thin skin, particularly on the ventral abdomen; tends to wrinkle (Fig. 41)
- easy bruising due to the increased fragility of the dermal vasculature
- calcinosis cutis; most often occurs on the dorsum, gluteal and inguinal region; about 40% of cases
- comedones
- secondary pyoderma
- poor wound healing
- seborrhoea sicca

Diagnosis

- history
- physical examination
- laboratory investigations

Laboratory findings

GENERAL
Routine haematology

This may reveal:
- eosinopenia (< 200 cells/m^3)
- lymphopenia (< 1200 lymphocytes/m^3)
- neutrophilia
- monocytosis
- erythrocytosis

Urinalysis
- low specific gravity (< 1.012)
- may be proteinuria
- bacteriuria in some cases
- glucose, if diabetes is a complicating factor

Biochemistry

This may reveal:
- elevated cholesterol (usually > 8 nmol/l)
- elevation of liver enzymes, particularly alkaline phosphatase, but also alanine transferase
- increased retention of bromsulphthalein (BSP)
- increased blood glucose, usually in the high normal range
- some cases (about 10%) may develop diabetes mellitus
- decreased levels of T4 due to excessive glucocorticoid levels (TSH response is normal)

SPECIFIC TESTS
ACTH response test

- starve the dog
- collect a plasma sample in the morning for cortisol measurement
- inject 10 units of ACTH gel intramuscularly (Synacthen, Ciba-Geigy) for a dog weighing less than 9 kg, or 20 units for a dog weighing more than 9 kg (0.8 ml Synacthen = 20 units ACTH gel)
- resample after 2 hours

In normal dogs the post-ACTH concentration of plasma cortisol is two to three times higher than basal levels. In the majority of dogs with pituitary-dependent hyperadrenocorticism, and in approximately half the adrenal tumour cases, there is an exaggerated response to ACTH stimulation (post-ACTH plasma cortisol levels greater than three times the basal level).

Low-dose
dexamethasone

As with the ACTH response test, the low-dose dexamethasone test is a useful screening test for the diagnosis of hyperadrenocorticism.

suppression test   The test is based on the fact that low doses of dexamethasone, in normal dogs, inhibit the release of pituitary ACTH, resulting in a decrease in the level of plasma cortisol. In dogs with hyperadrenocorticism, plasma cortisol levels are not markedly suppressed. The protocol is:

- starve the dog
- collect morning plasma sample for cortisol measurement
- inject 0.01 mg/kg dexamethasone intravenously
- collect further samples after 3 and 8 hours

High-dose   This test is based on the fact that high doses of dexamethasone will
dexamethasone   not suppress cortisol levels in dogs with adrenal tumours. The high
suppression test   levels of cortisol in these cases will have already suppressed ACTH. High levels of dexamethasone can, however, suppress ACTH secretion in dogs with pituitary-dependent hyperadrenocorticism. The protocol is:

- starve the dog
- collect plasma sample for cortisol measurement
- inject 0.1 mg/kg dexamethasone intravenously
- collect further plasma sample 3 and 8 hours later

If suppression of cortisol levels occurs, this is indicative of pituitary-dependent hyperadrenocorticism. Little or no suppression occurs in adrenal tumour cases.

Whichever method is used, it is necessary to contact the laboratory undertaking measurements since variations exist on the protocols described above, and it is therefore advisable to follow the recommended procedures of the laboratory in question.

Differential diagnosis

- during the early stages of the disease the differential diagnosis is that of any disease presenting as polydipsia and polyuria, for example, chronic renal disease
- once alopecia develops, the differential diagnosis includes:
  hypothyroidism
  Sertoli's cell tumour
  male feminizing syndrome
  ovarian imbalances

Treatment

SURGICAL   • bilateral adrenalectomy has been used as a treatment for pituitary-dependent hyperadrenocorticism. It requires experienced surgeons, and involves considerable risk to the dog. If successful, lifelong

treatment for hypoadrenocorticism will be necessary
- unilateral adrenalectomy is the treatment of choice for adrenal tumour. The surgery is difficult and should only be performed by experienced surgeons
- approximately half the adrenal tumours are carcinomas, metastasis being principally to the liver
- hypophysectomy has been reported as a treatment for pituitary-dependent hyperadrenocorticism. The surgery is extremely complex and is of academic interest only

MEDICAL
- most cases can be satisfactorily treated with o, p'-DDD (Mitotane, Idis Ltd). This drug, a chlorinated hydrocarbon related to DDT, selectively causes necrosis of the zona reticularis and zona fasciculata of the adrenal cortex. The mineralocorticoid-producing zona glomerulosa is relatively resistant in correctly dosed dogs

Method
- 50 mg/kg of mitotane is given daily by mouth with food until polydipsia stops (when the water intake drops to 60 ml/kg per day or less), or until lymphocyte counts return to 1000/mm^3. Alternatively, periodic ACTH tests can be performed and the daily dose of mitotane stopped when both pre- and post-ACTH stimulation levels of cortisol levels are below 200 nmol/l (Herrtage 1990). This is usually only necessary if the dog does not present initially with polydipsia
- the dog is then given a maintenance dose of 50 mg/kg weekly for the remainder of its life. If side-effects occur, half the maintenance dose given twice weekly may be helpful
- most dogs commence weekly therapy within a month with an average of 10 days, but each case is individual and careful monitoring is essential

Side-effects of mitotane
- vomiting (may occur within first few days due to gastric irritation). Giving in divided doses with food may help
- diarrhoea
- anorexia
- weakness, lethargy, depression

Feline hyperadrenocorticism

- hyperadrenocorticism is extremely rare in the cat. In those cases reported the signs were essentially the same as in the dog
- mitotane is unsuitable for therapy as the cat cannot tolerate this drug
- adrenalectomy is the treatment of choice for unilateral tumours of

the adrenal gland, and bilateral adrenalectomy may be tried on pituitary-dependent hyperadrenocorticism. The surgery is complex and should only be performed by experienced surgeons

SERTOLI'S CELL TUMOUR

• the most common testicular-related cause of skin disease
• any breed, but particularly boxer, Shetland sheepdog, poodle, Weimaraner, cairn terrier, Pekingese, collie and miniature schnauzer
• usually middle-aged to older dogs
• there is considerably more risk of tumour development in cryptorchid testes
• approximately 10% of these tumours are malignant, metastasis occurring via the regional lymph nodes to many organs (principally the lungs and liver)
• changes occur due to the excessive secretion of oestrogen

Clinical features

• bilaterally symmetrical non-pruritic alopecia: begins in the perineal and genital regions and spreads to involve the ventral abdomen, chest and flanks (Fig. 42)
• hyperpigmentation may occur with later lichenification and hyperkeratosis
• gynaecomastia
• preputial swelling
• in some cases there is a linear, well-demarcated area of erythema or, in more chronic cases, melanosis, along the ventral aspect of the prepuce
• decreased libido, may adopt the female squatting posture during urination and be sexually attractive to other dogs
• aspermatogenesis
• prostatic metaplasia
• the non-neoplastic testicle frequently atrophies
• in advanced cases there is a risk of bone marrow depression due to high levels of oestrogen

Diagnosis

• history
• physical examination
• radiography (abdominal testicle)
• histopathology of affected testicle
• elevated plasma oestrogen concentration

Differential diagnosis

- hypothyroidism
- hyperadrenocorticism
- idiopathic feminizing syndrome of male dogs
- growth hormone-responsive dermatosis
- castration-responsive alopecia

Treatment

- castration, both testes: check for metastasis clinically and radiographically prior to surgery
- response is usually seen in successful cases within 3 months; gynaecomastia is irreversible

MALE FEMINIZING SYNDROME

- unknown aetiology
- uncommon
- entire male dogs, any breed, middle to old age

Clinical features

Similar to Sertoli's cell tumour except:
- usually severe secondary seborrhoea, which may cause pruritus
- hyperpigmentation is more intense
- usually a ceruminous otitis is present
- testicles are normal (by physical and histopathological examination)
- hormonal assays are unhelpful

Treatment

- castration is effective in many cases
- response may take 3 months or more

TESTOSTERONE-RESPONSIVE ALOPECIA OF THE MALE DOG

- rare
- aetiology unknown (not proved hypoandrogenism)
- middle-aged to older dogs, any breed
- bilaterally symmetrical alopecia
- some cases have been castrated at an early age, others have cryptorchid, neoplastic or atrophied testicles; some dogs have apparently normal testicles

Diagnosis

- physical examination
- rule out differential diagnoses
- response to therapy

Differential diagnosis

- Sertoli's cell tumour
- hypothyroidism
- hyperadrenocorticism

Treatment

- methyltestosterone 1 mg/kg every other day (maximum total dose 30 mg)
- response should occur within 3 months
- maintenance dose once weekly
- risk of increased aggression and liver disease with testosterone therapy

CASTRATION-RESPONSIVE DERMATOSIS

- occurs in adult entire male dogs
- Pomeranian, chow-chow and keeshond may be predisposed
- the cause is poorly understood

Clinical features

- affected dogs develop a fine 'fluffy' coat with subsequent alopecia. In chronic states there may be hyperpigmentation

Diagnosis

- history
- physical examination
- rule out other endocrine disorders
- histopathological findings. These are similar to those seen in growth hormone-responsive dermatosis, including hair growth at biopsy sites, suggesting that some cases may represent a crossover syndrome

Treatment

- castration is curative, although testicular abnormalities are not present

PANHYPOPITUITARISM (PITUITARY DWARFISM)

• hereditary, thought to be autosomal recessive
• German shepherd dog and carnelian bear dog are predisposed
• most dogs have a cyst (Rathke's cyst) in the pituitary gland
• signs are principally related to lack of growth hormone, but there are others if the thyroid, adrenal or gonadal releasing hormones are deficient

Clinical features

• pups are normal until approximately 3 months of age, but subsequently fail to grow
• the puppy coat is retained and no primary hairs develop; hair is easily epilated
• bilaterally symmetrical alopecia gradually develops during the first year of life
• although short of stature, affected pups have virtually normal body proportions
• hyperpigmentation usually develops in the alopecic areas
• there may be other signs attributable to hypothyroidism or hypoadrenocorticism
• other abnormalities which may be noted include aggression (fear biting), short mandible, delayed dental eruption, cardiac disorders, megalo-oesophagus and gonadal abnormalities
• lifespan is often reduced

Diagnosis

• history
• physical examination and comparison with litter mates
• rule out other endocrine disorders
• biopsy: histopathology is that of a typical endocrinopathy — hyperkeratosis, follicular atrophy of the sebaceous glands, melanosis and thinning of the dermis; there is usually a decrease in the amount of dermal elastin
• radiography may reveal failure of the epiphyseal lines to close by the time the dog is adult
• growth stimulation tests show failure of growth hormone response

Differential diagnosis

• congenital hypothyroidism
• other congenital disease — renal, heart, gonadal defects
• juvenile diabetes mellitus

- malnutrition/malabsorption
- portal caval shunts

Treatment

- specific treatment for thyroid, adrenocortical or gonadal abnormalities if present
- growth hormone (difficult to obtain, expensive, may induce diabetes)
- response may take up to 3 months
- growth plates close rapidly and there is no appreciable increase in size

GROWTH HORMONE-RESPONSIVE DERMATOSIS (ADULT-ONSET HYPOSOMATOTROPISM, PSEUDO-CUSHING'S DISEASE)

- rare
- predominantly male, mature dogs with a breed disposition for — chow-chow, keeshond, Pomeranian and miniature poodle
- usual age of onset is 1−2 years
- cause is unknown

Clinical features

- bilaterally symmetrical alopecia and hyperpigmentation, mainly on the trunk, neck, pinnae and medial thighs (Fig. 43)
- the dogs are otherwise clinically normal

Diagnosis

- history
- physical examination
- rule out other endocrine disorders
- biopsy: orthokeratotic hyperkeratosis, follicular keratosis, follicular dilatation, epidermal melanosis, sebaceous gland atrophy, thin dermis, and reduced amounts and size of dermal elastin fibres
- hair tends to grow back at the biopsy site
- response to therapy

Differential diagnosis

- hypothyroidism
- hyperadrenocorticism

- sex hormone 'imbalances'

Treatment

- no treatment if owner accepts that the dog is otherwise well
- growth hormone, as for pituitary dwarfism
- beneficial response occurs within 3 months

ACROMEGALY

- acromegaly is a chronic disease associated with persistent excessive growth hormone, leading to overgrowth of soft tissue and bone
- may be associated with injection of anterior pituitary extracts, pituitary tumours and, in some bitches, by the administration of progestogens
- any age, breed, more commonly in bitches

Clinical features

- inspiratory stridor (soft tissue increased in pharyngeal respiratory inlet)
- increased body and paw size
- thickened myxoedematous skin
- hypertrichosis
- polydipsia, polyphagia, panting

Diagnosis

- history
- physical examination
- high plasma growth hormone levels which are not suppressed by intravenous glucose (1 mg/kg)
- biopsy: histopathological findings are increased collagen and mucin with hyperplasia of the epidermis

Treatment

- none unless associated with progestogens, these cases benefiting from stopping the administration of the progestogens or ovariohysterectomy

CANINE OVARIAN IMBALANCES

- poorly understood conditions
- diagnosis is made on clinical grounds only

- there are two types

Type 1 (hyperoestrogenism)

- middle-aged to old bitches
- any breed
- may be associated with cystic ovaries or ovarian tumours

Clinical features

- bilaterally symmetrical alopecia in the perineal and genital areas, extending anteriorly (Fig. 44)
- the affected area often exhibits a secondary seborrhoea and in chronic cases lichenification
- enlarged vulva and nipples
- abnormalities of the oestrus cycle

Diagnosis

- physical examination
- rule out other differential diagnoses
- response to treatment

Differential diagnosis

- hypothyroidism
- hyperadrenocorticism
- contact dermatitis
- hormonal hypersensitivity
- disorders presenting as seborrhoea

Treatment

- ovariohysterectomy
- symptomatic treatment for seborrhoea
- allow 3–6 months before assessing the response

Type 2 (oestrogen-responsive dermatosis)

- rare
- usually seen in bitches spayed before the first oestrus
- cause is unknown; hypo-oestrogenism has not been demonstrated

Clinical features

- bilaterally symmetrical alopecia in the perineal and genital regions,

which spreads to the medial thighs and the ventral abdomen; the dorsum is spared
- the remaining coat tends to be soft, like that of a puppy; hair-shedding is minimal
- pruritus is minimal unless there is a secondary seborrhoea
- the vulva and nipples are small

Diagnosis

- physical examination
- rule out differential diagnoses
- response to treatment

Differential diagnosis

- hypothyroidism
- hyperadrenocorticism
- disorders presenting with seborrhoea

Treatment

- no treatment is necessary in many cases
- 0.1 − 1 mg/kg stilboestrol once daily by mouth for three weeks of each month
- thereafter maintenance dose of 0.1 − 1 mg weekly
- alternative non-stilbene oestrogens include oestradiol valerate (equal potency to stilboestrol) or ethinyloestradiol (20 times more potent)
- monitor the dogs due to risk of bone marrow depression and pancytopenia

DIABETES MELLITUS

- diabetes mellitus in dogs may be associated with skin lesions
- usually cutaneous lesions consist of pyoderma, seborrhoea, thin, hypotonic skin and alopecia

Hepatocutaneous syndrome

- rare
- dogs
- in four dogs reported by Walton and others (1986) cutaneous lesions consisted of an erythematous, ulcerative, crusting dermatosis, usually occurring on the face, genitals, distal extremities and footpads

- these lesions preceded the typical signs of diabetes mellitus and hepatic disease
- affected dogs may be predisposed to dermatophyte infections

Diagnosis

- history
- physical examination
- laboratory investigations
- biopsy

The condition resembles glucagonoma syndrome in humans (necrolytic migratory erythema). Most affected dogs have not presented with pancreatic tumours; hepatic cirrhosis has been the significant pathological abnormality.

Treatment

- the condition is resistant to treatment and the prognosis is poor

FELINE SYMMETRIC ALOPECIA (FELINE ENDOCRINE ALOPECIA)

- this is a condition of multiple aetiology
- a precise endocrine cause has not been documented, hence the previous term endocrine alopecia is no longer in favour

Clinical features

- any sex or breed
- neutered males (90%) and females
- bilaterally symmetrical alopecia of the perineal and genital regions extending to the ventral abdomen, thighs and tail, and in advanced cases the flank and front limbs. The dorsal region is unaffected (Fig. 45)
- non-pruritic
- in all other respects the cats are normal

Diagnosis

- history
- examination of shed hairs microscopically to assess whether the hairs have been broken off (chewing/licking) or have been shed (intact, pointed hairs)
- physical examination
- rule out differential diagnoses
- response to therapy

Differential diagnosis

- flea-bite hypersensitivity
- dermatophyte infection
- psychogenic alopecia
- telogen defluxion
- demodicosis (rare, but all cases should have skin scrapings)

Treatment

- treatment is empirical, most cases responding to one of the methods described below
- adequate time must be allowed for hair regrowth — up to 3 months

THYROID TREATMENT

At least some cats may have low functional reserve (Thoday 1986) and 80% of cats will respond to thyroid treatment.
- 100 µg/day of L-triiodothyronine (Tertroxin, Coopers Pitman-Moore) is given in divided doses; once hair growth has occurred lower doses may be given for maintenance

PROGESTOGEN TREATMENT

- megestrol acetate (Ovarid, Coopers Pitman-Moore) is given at a dose of 5 mg twice weekly. Side-effects may be seen and these are described under miliary dermatitis (pp. 166–167)
- an alternative drug is proligesterone (Delvosterone, Mycofarm). 100 mg is given subcutaneously. This dose may be repeated in 4 months depending on the response

SEX HORMONE TREATMENT

- some cases in either sex respond to an injection of testosterone phenylpropionate (Androjet, Intervet). The advised dose is 5 mg. Undesirable virilization may occur in some individuals
- some authorities maintain that a combination of androgen/oestrogen therapy gives better results

7/Physical and Chemical Skin Disease

NASAL SOLAR DERMATITIS

- phototoxic reaction
- tends to occur in unpigmented skin, particularly of the nose, but may also be seen on the eyelids and lips any breed, sex or age
- caused by repeated exposure to ultraviolet light, and is therefore more common in warm sunny climates
- the condition is frequently seasonal in the early stages, with increasing severity as time passes

Clinical features

- erythema and alopecia of the planum nasale
- later crusting, ulceration and exudation
- in chronic untreated cases there is a risk of the development of squamous cell carcinoma, with rapid nasal erosion

Diagnosis

- history
- physical examination
- response to treatment
- skin biopsy — may develop squamous cell carcinoma

Differential diagnosis

- discoid lupus erythematosus
- systemic lupus erythematosus
- pemphigus erythematosus
- pemphigus foliaceus
- nasal pyoderma
- dermatophyte infection
- dermatomyositis
- contact hypersensitivity (plastic food dish)

Treatment

- avoid sunlight
- topical glucocorticoids
- sunscreen agents which contain *para*-aminobenzoic acid (PABA)

may be rubbed into the nose
- tattooing with black ink

FELINE SOLAR DERMATITIS

- any age, breed or sex
- most commonly seen in white cats, or cats with white ears
- mainly a condition of warm, sunny climates, but cases are seen in old cats in temperate climates

Clinical features

- initially there is erythema of the margin of the pinna
- each summer there is a deterioration so that the condition progresses from erythema to skin peeling, crusting and self-excoriation
- in white blue-eyed cats, the margin of the lower eyelids may be affected
- in chronic cases a squamous cell carcinoma may develop which is destructive to the pinna, although metastasis is rare (Fig. 46)

Diagnosis

- history
- physical examination
- biopsy: squamous cell carcinoma?

Differential diagnosis

- ear mite infestation
- fight wounds
- feline scabies
- frost-bite
- pemphigus foliaceus
- systemic lupus erythematosus
- cold agglutinin disease

Treatment

- avoid sunlight
- glucocorticoid creams
- capsules containing a carotenoid (110 mg β-carotene and 150 mg canthaxanthin) may be beneficial
- cosmetic surgery to remove part of the pinna; hair regrowth protects the underlying skin from further ultraviolet ray damage

- surgical excision of the pinna is the only effective treatment for squamous cell carcinoma; cosmetic results are usually very satisfactory

SOLAR DERMATITIS OF THE TRUNK

- dogs
- predisposed breeds include the Dalmatian and English bull-terriers
- seen in warm sunny climates

Clinical features

- early lesions are erythema and scaling
- these lesions occur principally on the trunk and abdomen, in dogs that are allowed outside without access to shade or dogs that habitually sunbathe
- after a few years the skin may become thicker, with erosions, ulceration and secondary infection
- finally, some dogs develop squamous cell carcinoma

Treatment

- the most practical measure is to keep the dog out of sunlight for as much time as possible from an early stage

PRIMARY IRRITANT CONTACT DERMATITIS

- must be differentiated from contact hypersensitivity
- primary irritant dermatitis is more common than contact hypersensitivity
- there are a very large variety of substances capable of causing irritation. These are divided into absolute and relative types: absolute types include acids and alkalis that are universally irritant in all dogs and cats; relative types include soaps, detergents and solvents, and inert substances such as gravel and sand. Flea collars, especially if fitted too tightly, have also caused irritation

Clinical features

- lesions are erythema, papules, crusts and excoriation
- common sites are the ventral surface of the abdomen, axilla, interdigital space, perineum, scrotum and any other area where hair is sparse

• hairy skin is relatively unaffected unless the irritant is a shampoo or spray

Diagnosis

• history — most important
• physical examination
• elimination and provocative exposure tests

Differential diagnosis

• atopy
• contact hypersensitivity
• food hypersensitivity
• staphylococcal folliculitis
• seborrhoea
• scabies
• dermatophyte infection
• solar dermatitis
• drug eruption

Treatment

• history — find the irritant substance and remove it
• bathing and topical glucocorticoid ointments give temporary symptomatic relief

BURNS

• burns may be divided into full-thickness and partial-thickness
• full-thickness burns involve the complete destruction of the epidermis and adnexa; with healing there is migration of epithelial cells from the edge of the burn
• partial-thickness burns involve incomplete destruction of the epidermis, and re-epithelialization is possible
• secondary pyoderma is common

Clinical features

• causes include boiling water, fat, infra-red lamps, hair-driers and hot-water bottles
• initially there is pain at the site of the burn, then after a day or so the skin over the affected area becomes dry and hard
• later there is secondary infection, the skin becomes necrotic and may slough

- if more than 25% of the body surface is involved, the animal will be systemically ill

Diagnosis

- history
- physical examination

Treatment

- remove necrotic tissue
- gentle bathing and cleaning
- topical antibacterial ointments
- fluid therapy and plasma or plasma expanders for severely ill animals

FROST-BITE

- severe cold conditions ($-30°C$), when dogs and cats are left outside for prolonged periods
- rare in healthy animals accustomed to the cold, more likely in sick animals, and in those that have recently moved to a cold climate from a warm one
- the commonest sites are the tips of the tail and ears in cats, and the scrotum in male dogs

Clinical features

- alopecia, erythema, scaliness at predisposed sites
- loss of pigmentation
- later there may be necrosis and sloughing of affected areas

Diagnosis

- history
- physical examination

Treatment

- thaw rapidly in warm water; do not attempt to do this outside or the affected area may refreeze and make matters worse
- topical antibacterial creams
- surgical debridement; wait until there is a clear demarcation between healthy and necrotic tissue

8/Immunological Skin Disease

HYPERSENSITIVITY SKIN DISORDERS

Clinical hypersensitivity disorders have been classified by Gel and Coombes. The following description is simplified since in many instances complex interactions occur simultaneously.

Type 1 (immediate, anaphylactic)

• genetically susceptible individuals inhale (absorb percutaneously?) allergens such as pollen and house dust, and produce immuno-globulin E (IgE), which fixes to tissue mast cells and blood basophils
• the allergen subsequently comes into contact with its specific IgE, leading to the release of vasoactive amines, which cause tissue damage
• examples are urticaria, angio-oedema, atopy, drug eruption and flea-bite hypersensitivity

Type 2 (cytotoxic)

• IgG or IgM with or without complement binds to complete antigens on body tissues
• the antigen–antibody reaction causes cell lysis
• examples are pemphigus, pemphigoid, cold agglutinin disease and drug eruption

Type 3 (immune complex)

• circulating antigen–antibody complexes fix complement and are deposited in blood vessel walls
• these complexes attract neutrophils; proteolytic and hydrolytic enzymes released from the neutrophils produce tissue damage
• examples are systemic lupus erythematosus and bacterial hypersensitivity

Type 4 (delayed)

• incomplete allergen (hapten) combines with tissue protein, e.g. collagen; this complete allergen is processed by monocytes, macro-phages or Langerhans cells and sensitizes T-lymphocytes

- sensitized T-lymphocytes respond to subsequent challenge by releasing lymphokines, which produce tissue damage
- an example is contact hypersensitivity

Urticaria (hives)

- seen in dogs and cats
- uncommon
- type 1 and 3
- many possible causes — e.g. drugs, vaccines, insect bites or stings, infections

Clinical features

- acute onset
- localized or generalized wheals
- hair in affected lesions stands up
- variable pruritus

Diagnosis

- history
- physical examination
- investigation of possible underlying causes

Differential diagnosis

- superficial folliculitis
- cutaneous neoplasia
- dermatophyte infection
- demodicosis

Treatment

- establish the underlying cause if possible and remove it
- glucocorticoids given systemically — drug of choice is prednisolone at a dose of 2 mg/kg for a few days

Angio-oedema (angioneurotic oedema)

- dogs and cats
- type 1 hypersensitivity
- commonly due to wasp and bee stings, but other causes as for urticaria
- cutaneous response is more dramatic than with urticaria, with extreme swelling of the face, head or feet

- laryngeal oedema may occur

Diagnosis

- history (e.g. seen playing with a wasp)
- physical examination

Treatment

- elimination of known cause
- adrenaline 1:1000, 0.1−0.5 ml subcutaneously
- glucocorticoid therapy as for urticaria — intravenous route preferred
- consider tracheotomy if severe laryngeal oedema

Atopy (atopic disease)

- defined as an inherited predisposition to develop IgE antibodies to environmental allergens resulting in allergic disease (Halliwell & Gorman, 1989)
- common
- occurs in dogs and cats
- many allergens may be responsible, including:
  house dust
  house dust mite
  human dander
  animal dander
  pollens
  fungi
  moulds
  feathers

Canine atopy

- any breed, including crossbreeds; certain breeds are predisposed. These include West Highland white, cairn terrier, Scottish terrier, Dalmatian, English setter, pug, boxer, Boston terrier, Lhasa apso, wire-haired fox terrier and miniature schnauzer. Breed disposition may alter both geographically and in time, since if an atopic dog attains champion status in the show ring it is likely that there will be an increased incidence in that breed as the dog is used at stud

Clinical features

- most cases begin symptoms between 1 and 3 years of age with a range of 6 months to 7 years

• clinical signs may be seasonal at first but many dogs develop hypersensitivity to further allergens and symptoms then persist all year round. Other dogs have a history of non-seasonal symptoms from the start
• pruritus is the principal complaint
• typically the sites affected are the face, the ventrum and axilla, and the feet (Figs 47–49)
• there may be erythema, but most lesions seen are secondary; these consist of pyoderma, seborrhoea, lichenification (in more chronic cases) and alopecia. Self-trauma is common and may confuse the clinical picture
• other features which may be seen include salivary staining of the coat as a result of constant licking, conjunctivitis, otitis externa and hyperhidrosis (sweating)

Diagnostic procedures

INTRADERMAL ALLERGY TESTING

• in order to minimize poor results it is important to select cases carefully prior to performing intradermal testing; an intelligent, co-operative owner aware of the complexities of investigation is also useful

Pre-testing investigations

• history and physical examination should suggest atopy; do not test every pruritic dog without a careful history and physical examination
• rule out parasitic involvement, particularly scabies and fleas. Although atopic dogs are predisposed to develop flea-bite hypersensitivity, if fleas are present these should be eliminated prior to performing intradermal testing so that the relative importance of the fleas in inducing pruritus can be ascertained. If there is any doubt at all concerning scabies, a therapeutic trial is useful before proceeding any further. Such procedures also allow time for any glucocorticoids which may have been previously administered to be eliminated from the system
• seborrhoea and pyoderma are treated to ensure that they are not the primary cause of the pruritus. If pruritus ceases with proper treatment of pyoderma and seborrhoea, it is unlikely that atopy is an underlying cause and another line of investigation will be needed
• dietary investigations are routinely performed prior to skin testing to rule out food hypersensitivity (p. 98)
• ensure that no anti-inflammatory drugs have been administered recently. It is difficult to make precise recommendations as to how long to wait prior to testing. This will depend on the length of time glucocorticoids have been given. If repositol glucocorticoids have been used, there may be a wait of some months before positive reactions will occur. For this reason and for others discussed else-

where in this book, repositol glucocorticoids are to be avoided in the management of pruritic skin conditions in the dog

Allergen selection
- consult with physicians to determine what allergens are common in the locality
- use standardized veterinary *aqueous* allergens only; these are currently not available in the United Kingdom. Reliable allergens are available from HAL Laboratories (Haarlem, Holland) or Greer Laboratories (Lenior, N.C., USA)

Technique of intradermal allergy testing
- the dog is placed in lateral recumbency and the hair of the flank is carefully clipped. Xylazine hydrochloride (Rompun, Bayer, UK) 0.45 mg/kg intravenously with 0.04 mg/kg atropine sulphate subcutaneously is used for sedation except in calm individuals. Other sedatives are not indicated as they will interfere with reactions
- a felt-tipped pen is used to mark each injection site
- 0.05 ml of each test allergen is injected *intradermally*, using a 26-gauge needle. A positive control injection (0.05 ml of 1:100000 histamine phosphate) and negative control (0.05 ml of diluent) is also injected
- the injection sites are examined 15 and 30 minutes later
- a positive reaction is a wheal equal to or larger in diameter than the difference between the positive and negative controls (Fig. 50)
- positive reactions should be compared with the allergens known to be in the dog's environment as established in the history
- there are many pitfalls associated with allergy testing and both false positive and false negative reactions may occur
- the commonest causes of false positive reactions are irritant allergens containing glycerine, trauma with too large a needle, injection of irritant contaminants, injection of too large a volume, and injecting into already inflamed skin
- some causes of false negative reactions include subcutaneous injection, using too-weak allergens (out of date, mixes), and interference from previously administered glucocorticoids or antihistamines

RADIOALLERGO-
SORBENT TEST
- the radioallergosorbent test (RAST) is an *in vitro* test which has recently become available commercially in the USA
- RAST measures the concentration of canine allergen-specific IgE in serum
- correlation with intradermal testing is variable, in some instances being good and in others poor. In addition high levels of background IgE may limit the usefulness of the test. Refinement of the test in the future may greatly increase its value, although at the time of writing most authorities prefer intradermal allergy testing

Willemse (1986) has suggested major and minor features in order to clarify the diagnosis of atopy.

MAJOR FEATURES   At least three should be present:
- a breed predilection
- a familial history of atopy
- pruritus
- facial and/or digital involvement
- chronic or chronically relapsing dermatitis
- lichenification of the flexor surface of the tarsus or the extensor surface of the carpus

MINOR FEATURES   At least three should be present:
- onset before 3 years of age
- conjunctivitis
- facial erythema and cheilitis
- superficial pyoderma
- hyperhidrosis
- positive intradermal allergy testing
- elevated allergen-specific IgE
- elevated allergen-specific IgGd

Differential diagnosis

- flea-bite hypersensitivity
- food hypersensitivity
- contact hypersensitivity
- scabies
- other diseases leading to secondary pyoderma
- hookworm dermatitis
- subcorneal pustular dermatitis

Treatment

- avoidance of allergens is occasionally beneficial if only one or two allergens are involved, for example exclude from the bedroom in dust hypersensitivity
- *systemic glucocorticoids*: prednisolone is the drug of choice. It must be given on alternate days, thus minimizing the risk of adrenal cortex suppression. Therapy is lifelong
- *antihistamines*: these drugs are not particularly effective but their trial use is warranted, since some cases benefit. Various antihistamines should be tried, as some cases will respond to one type while others respond to a different drug
- *hyposensitization*: repeated injections of initially increasing amounts of allergen are given in an attempt to modify the immune response. The mode of action is unclear, but placebo-controlled double-blind trials have demonstrated their effectiveness (Willemse and others 1984). A satisfactory response may take up to 9 months, and

definitive conclusions as to effectiveness in any one particular case should not be made before this time. It is therefore important to pick cases and owners carefully and explain procedures in detail before attempting hyposensitization in order to maximize the possibility of success

- low-dose alternate-day prednisolone may be used in conjunction with hyposensitization in severe cases
- approximately 50% of atopic dogs benefit to some extent from hyposensitization in that either glucocorticoid therapy is no longer needed or a reduced dose will control symptoms
- *essential fatty acid supplementation* (EFAs)
- EFAs have recently become available in the UK (Efavet, Efamol) for the treatment of atopy. These substances have been shown to modify inflammation by promoting anti-inflammatory prostaglandins and inhibiting the production of pro-inflammatory substances such as thromboxanes and leucotrienes. Some cases, but not all, are controlled well by the use of essential fatty acids, which thus offer a safe alternative to glucocorticoids

Feline atopy

- increasingly recognized world-wide including the UK

Clinical features

- seasonal or non-seasonal
- facial pruritus
- pruritic ears
- miliary dermatitis-like lesions
- indolent ('rodent') ulcer, eosinophilic plaque or granuloma
- symmetric alopecia
- generalized pruritus

Diagnosis

- history
- physical examination
- investigation of other causes of the clinical features listed
- intradermal allergy testing. Reactions tend to be more diffuse than in dogs and hence more difficult to interpret

Treatment

- prednisolone 2 mg/kg initially, then when control is achieved given on an alternate-day basis
- essential fatty acid supplementation (Efavet, Efamol). Preliminary

work suggests that this approach is promising, although controlled trials have not yet been performed in cats

Food hypersensitivity (food allergy)

- uncommon
- dogs and cats
- thought to involve type 1, 2 and 4 hypersensitivity reactions
- hypersensitivity usually develops to specific items in the diet, such as beef, fish, milk. Change of diet prior to the onset of symptoms is not significant since the allergen has frequently been a component of the animal's diet for months or years before the commencement of symptoms

Clinical features

- any age, sex, breed
- symptoms are variable, and the condition can mimic any dermatosis

DOGS
- pruritus
- pruritic superficial folliculitis
- seborrhoea
- urticaria

CATS
- miliary dermatitis-like lesions
- facial dermatitis (Fig. 51)
- generalized pruritus
- seborrhoea
- urticaria
- psychogenic alopecia
- indolent ulcer
- eosinophilic plaque/granuloma

Diagnosis

- history
- physical examination
- *dietary investigation*
- a detailed list is made of the animal's diet
- protein sources unfamiliar to the animal, such as cooked lamb or chicken plus rice, are fed to the exclusion of all other food for two weeks. Emphasize to the owner that all members of the family, including children, must understand that no other scraps of food must be given at this time
- improvement while on the hypoallergenic diet suggests food

hypersensitivity. Individual items are then added to the diet every week; relapse followed by remission when the food item is removed again identifies the allergen
- note that changing from one brand of commercial food to another is not helpful since the offending allergen is likely to be in both brands
- intradermal allergy testing is of *no value* in the diagnosis of food hypersensitivity

Differential diagnosis

DOGS
- atopy
- flea-bite hypersensitivity
- scabies
- superficial folliculitis
- pediculosis
- intestinal parasitic hypersensitivity
- seborrhoea
- drug hypersensitivity

CATS
- atopy
- flea-bite hypersensitivity
- cheyletiellosis
- pediculosis
- dermatophyte infection
- drug hypersensitivity
- intestinal parasitic hypersensitivity
- trombiculidiasis
- psychogenic alopecia

Treatment

- avoid the specific allergen in the diet
- if this is not identified, feed the hypoallergenic diet used to investigate the cause. This diet will need to be balanced with mineral and fatty acid supplements
- in both dogs and cats there is frequently a poor response to glucocorticoids

Contact hypersensitivity (allergic contact dermatitis)

- uncommon (primary irritant dermatitis more common)
- dogs and cats
- type 4 hypersensitivity
- many substances have been incriminated in contact hypersensitivity. Examples of allergens are:

pollens and resins
soaps
shampoos
topical ointments, especially those containing neomycin
insecticides
disinfectants
flea collars
wool, nylon fibre
dyes, mordants, finishes used in the manufacture of carpets and
    blankets
rubber and plastic

Clinical features

• hypersensitivity usually develops to a substance which the dog or
cat has been in contact with for at least 6 months. Hence a history
of recent change of bedding or carpets is *not* generally significant
• lesions occur in contact sites (Fig. 52): the ventral abdomen, feet,
scrotum, chin, neck and pinnae. If a plastic dish is involved lesions
occur around the mouth and nose
• lesions may be seasonal or non-seasonal and consist of erythema,
macules and papules in acute cases, and hyperpigmentation in
chronic cases. Self-trauma and secondary pyoderma are common
• pruritus varies from mild to extreme

Diagnosis

• history
• physical examination
• elimination and provocative exposure:
    the animal is kept away from suspect allergens for 2 weeks, for
        example kept off grass, or housed in the kitchen and not
        allowed in the rest of the house
• if there is contact hypersensitivity there is remission of clinical
signs followed by relapse when the animal comes back into contact
with the allergen. Individual items, such as carpets, bedding, are
exposed to the animal item by item for a week at a time. (Remember
that contact hypersensitivity is a delayed response, and that reactions will not occur in less than 48 hours)
• an intelligent co-operative owner is required for the above investigation or failure to identify the allergen will be inevitable

PATCH TESTING   Patch testing is theoretically the best method to diagnose contact
hypersensitivity and is the standard approach in man. In animals it

is difficult to get the animal's co-operation. Two methods have been advocated

Closed patch testing
- suspect allergens are placed in close contact with skin on the flank after clipping
- in order to facilitate close contact between the allergens and the skin, Finn chambers may be used. These are obtained from Associated Hospital Supplies (PO Box 4, Pershore, Worcestershire, UK). Finn chambers are shallow metal containers mounted on Scampor (non-woven microporous adhesive tape). The suspect allergen is placed in each chamber, and the supporting tape fixed to the flank by means of a body bandage
- Elizabethan collars may be needed to prevent interference by the animal
- the chambers are removed after 48 hours and the animal examined for positive reactions, which tend to be mild erythema. Doubtful cases are examined again at 72 hours

Open patch testing
- the test material is applied to the clipped skin and the solvent allowed to evaporate
- suggested allergen concentrations have been given by Walton (1977)
- the test site is examined after 48 hours, positive reactions showing as erythema

Differential diagnosis

- primary irritant contact dermatitis
- atopy
- food hypersensitivity
- scabies
- *Pelodera* dermatitis
- hookworm dermatitis
- superficial pyoderma

Treatment

- avoid the offending allergen
- glucocorticoids — response is variable and rarely totally satisfactory
- hyposensitization is *not* effective

Drug eruption

- rare

- cutaneous or mucocutaneous reaction to a drug
- dogs and cats
- thought to be associated with all types of hypersensitivity reactions
- the reaction may occur even though the drug has been administered long-term to the animal without previous problems, or it may occur after only a few days of administration

Clinical features

- lesions are very variable and may mimic virtually any dermatosis
- possible lesions include: papules, seborrhoea, vesicles, alopecia, ulceration, urticaria and otitis externa

Diagnosis

- history
- physical examination
- biopsy: perivascular dermatitis, subepidermal vesicular dermatitis, intraepidermal vesiculopustular dermatitis
- response to removal of the drug
- do *not* readminister the drug to determine whether a relapse occurs; this may provoke anaphylaxis

Differential diagnosis

- virtually any dermatosis

Treatment

- discontinue the offending drug and avoid drugs of the same group
- symptomatic therapy, bathing and antibacterial agents
- glucocorticoids are frequently not effective

Intestinal parasitic hypersensitivity

- uncommon
- dogs and cats
- immunology poorly understood; possibly involves type I hypersensitivity

Clinical features

- lesions are usually pruritic crusting papules or seborrhoea
- elimination of parasites is followed by recovery; relapse if reinfestation occurs

Diagnosis

- history
- physical examination
- faecal examination
- response to treatment

Treatment

- elimination of parasites

Hormonal hypersensitivity

- rare
- dogs
- immunology poorly understood; possibly type 1 and 4 reactions to progesterone, oestrogen or testosterone

Clinical features

- no breed or age predilection, but most cases reported in intact females
- pruritic, papulocrustous lesions of perineal, genital and thigh regions
- the lesions are bilaterally symmetrical and may spread to involve the feet, face and ears in advanced cases
- there may be enlargement of the nipples and vulva
- there are often irregular oestrus cycles or pseudopregnancy

Diagnosis

- history
- physical examination
- intradermal testing with aqueous progesterone (0.025 mg), oestrogen (0.0125 mg) or testosterone (0.05 mg). Check for immediate and delayed hypersensitivity reactions
- response to therapy

Differential diagnosis

- flea-bite hypersensitivity
- food hypersensitivity
- atopy
- folliculitis
- drug eruption
- ovarian imbalance type 1
- intestinal parasitic hypersensitivity

Treatment

• neuter
• female dogs may respond to testosterone, but this is only of use to reduce pruritus prior to ovariohysterectomy

Flea-bite hypersensitivity

This is discussed under parasitic conditions (pp. 28–29).

AUTOIMMUNE DISORDERS

Pemphigus complex

• the pemphigus complex comprises a group of *rare* autoimmune diseases described in dogs and cats
• the diseases are vesiculobullous ulcerative disorders of the skin and often the mucous membranes
• autoantibody is directed against the epidermal intercellular cement substance and may be demonstrated by direct immunofluorescence testing
• histologically the pemphigus complex is characterized by acantholysis (loss of cohesion between individual epidermal cells)

Pemphigus foliaceus

• the most common of the autoimmune diseases
• dogs and cats
• no age, breed or sex predisposition

Clinical features

• often begins on the face, nose and ears as a vesiculobullous or exfoliative pustular dermatitis (Figs 53 and 54)
• footpads are frequently involved with hyperkeratosis
• mucocutaneous lesions are uncommon

Diagnosis

• history
• physical examination
• histological examination: subcorneal acantholysis leading to the development of a cleft. Within the cleft there are neutrophils and eosinophils
• direct immunofluorescence may reveal intercellular deposition of immunoglobulin throughout the epidermis

Differential diagnosis

- bacterial folliculitis
- dermatophyte infection
- seborrhoea
- systemic lupus erythematosus
- discoid lupus erythematosus
- subcorneal pustular dermatosis
- zinc-responsive dermatosis
- dermatomyositis
- neoplasia

Treatment

- glucocorticoids are key drugs and prednisolone is the drug of choice. The dose suggested (Scott *et al.* 1987) is 4.4 mg/kg orally, which may cause unacceptable polyphagia, polydipsia and polyuria
- in order to reduce these side-effects the following combination protocols are suggested:
    glucocorticoid therapy and gold salt therapy (chrysotherapy) may be more successful in some cases (Fig. 55). Aurothioglucose (Solganol, Schering) or sodium aurothiomalate (Myocrisin, May and Baker) is given at a test dose of 1 mg intramuscularly initially, then 2 mg a week later; subsequently 1 mg/kg at weekly intervals
    the addition of chrysotherapy may permit lower doses of glucocorticoids or abolish their need altogether
    glucocorticoids and azathioprine (Imuran, Wellcome). Azathioprine is given at a dose of 2 mg/kg once daily and then on alternate days. When remission is achieved, it may be possible to reduce the dose of prednisolone, gradually phasing it out completely while maintaining the azathioprine
- azathioprine is not recommended in cats
- side-effects may occur with the above therapy (principally blood dyscrasias) and therefore complete blood counts and platelet counts are recommended at monthly intervals
- without treatment the prognosis is poor. With treatment the prognosis is fair

Pemphigus vulgaris

- dogs and cats
- no age, breed or sex predisposition
- the most severe form

Clinical features

DOGS
- vesiculobullous, ulcerative, erosive lesions of the oral mucosa and mucocutaneous junctions (lips, nose, eyelids, prepuce, vulva, anus) and the skin (particularly the axilla and the groin). There may be involvement of the nail-bed, leading to onychomadesis
- oral cavity lesions occur in approximately 90% of dogs
- intact bullae are rarely seen due to the thin epidermis and self-trauma
- the dog may be anorexic, depressed or febrile

CATS
- vesiculobullous disorder of the oral mucocutaneous junction, involving the lips, hard palate, gums and planum nasale

Diagnosis

- history
- physical examination
- biopsy; acantholysis occurs just above the stratum germinativum of the epidermis, leading to cleft formation. The basal epidermal cells adhere to the basement membrane ('tombstones')
- Nikolsky sign: digital pressure can slip the epidermis
- immunofluorescence: positive for IgG, occasionally complement within the epidermis
- direct smears from intact vesicles or recent erosions may show numerous acantholytic keratinocytes

Differential diagnosis

- bullous pemphigoid
- drug eruption
- systemic lupus erythematosus
- mycosis fungoides
- toxic epidermal necrolysis
- erythema multiforme
- candidiasis
- other causes of stomatitis

Treatment

- as discussed under pemphigus foliaceus
- often fatal unless treated

Pemphigus erythematosus

- dogs and cats

- no age, breed or sex predilection
- may be a benign form of pemphigus foliaceus

Clinical features

- similar to pemphigus foliaceus but localized to the head and neck
- there may be nasal depigmentation with resultant secondary photodermatitis

Diagnosis, differential diagnosis and treatment

This is as for pemphigus foliaceus.

Pemphigus vegetans

- dogs
- least common form — extremely rare
- no age, breed or sex predisposition
- may be a benign form of pemphigus vulgaris

Clinical features

- verrucous vegetation and papillomatous proliferation, especially over the dorsum and trunk

Diagnosis and treatment

This is as for pemphigus foliaceus.

Bullous pemphigoid

- dogs
- no age or sex predilection but collies, Shetland sheepdogs and Dobermanns may be predisposed

Clinical features

- vesiculobullous lesions that may affect the oral cavity, mucocutaneous junctions or skin
- about 80% of dogs have oral lesions
- cutaneous lesions occur most commonly in the axillae or groin
- there may paronychia, ulceration of the pads or onychomadesis
- severely affected dogs may be anorexic, febrile and depressed and clinically indistinguishable from pemphigus vulgaris

Diagnosis

• history
• physical examination
• biopsy: subepidermal cleft and vesicle formation
• immunofluorescence: positive IgG, IgM or IgA and usually complement (C3) at the basement membrane zone
• the above tests should be performed on intact vesicles or bullae, and it may be necessary to hospitalize the dog to wait for the development of these lesions, as they are transient
• microscopic examination of direct smears from intact vesicles or bullae does not reveal acantholytic keratinocytes

Treatment

• as for pemphigus foliaceus
• prognosis guarded, may be fatal without treatment. Other cases appear relatively benign and localized

Cold agglutinin disease

• dogs and cats
• rare
• associated with cold-reacting erythrocyte antibodies (especially IgM), which are most active at 0−4°C
• type 2 hypersensitivity
• most cases are idiopathic, some cases in dogs have been associated with lead poisoning and in cats with upper respiratory infections

Clinical features

• erythema, purpura, necrosis and ulceration
• sites affected include the paws, tips of the ears and tail, and the nose
• lesions are exacerbated by cold

Diagnosis

• history
• physical examination
• Coombs' test at 4°C using reagent with activity against IgM
• autohaemagglutination of blood on a slide may occur if the blood is cooled from room temperature to 0°C. This reaction is reversible on warming the slide to 37°C

Differential diagnosis

- dermatomyositis
- vasculitis
- frost-bite
- disseminated intravascular coagulation
- systemic lupus erythematosus

Treatment

- correction of the underlying cause if possible
- immunosuppressive drugs such as glucocorticoids or azathioprine
- avoid cold

Discoid lupus erythematosus

- dogs
- uncommon; affects principally the nose and other parts of the face
- reported in collies, German shepherd dogs, Shetland sheepdogs and Siberian huskies
- no age or sex predilection

Clinical features

- early lesions are depigmentation, erythema and scaling of the planum nasale (Fig. 56)
- subsequently there may be crusting, erosive or ulcerative lesions which spread to the bridge of the nose, and less frequently the periorbital region, ears and distal limbs
- the condition is exacerbated by sunlight

Diagnosis

- history
- physical examination
- biopsy: hydropic or lichenoid interface dermatitis, with hydropic degeneration, lymphocytic infiltration and thickening of the basement membrane zone
- direct immunofluorescence: deposition of immunoglobulin or complement or both at the basement membrane zone

Differential diagnosis

- demodicosis

- dermatophyte infection
- nasal pyoderma
- pemphigus foliaceus
- pemphigus erythematosus
- subcorneal pustular dermatosis
- dermatomyositis
- contact hypersensitivity
- Vogt−Koyanagi−Harada-like syndrome

Treatment

- avoid sunlight
- prednisolone 1 mg/kg orally b.i.d.
- vitamin E 400 IU b.i.d. orally
- vitamin E may be used in conjunction with glucocorticoids. It has a 4- to 8-week lag period before clinical benefit

Systemic lupus erythematosus

- uncommon
- dogs and cats
- autoantibodies are directed against many tissues
- the pathogenesis is unclear; there may be genetic, infective, immunological (lack of suppressor T-cell activity), endocrine and drug factors. Drugs such as chlorpromazine, hydralazine, isoniazid and phenytoin may be implicated
- sunlight exacerbates the cutaneous lesions
- no age or sex predilections in dogs or cats
- in dogs, the collie, Shetland sheepdog and German shepherd dog may be predisposed

Clinical features

- non-cutaneous; possibilities include:
  polyarthritis
  glomerulonephritis
  pyrexia
  anaemia
  peripheral lymphadenopathy
  oral ulceration
  pericarditis
  polymyositis
  pleuritis
  neurological disorders
- cutaneous; diverse possibilities include:

mucocutaneous ulcerative lesions
alopecia
seborrhoea
refractory pyoderma
facial dermatitis
footpad lesions (ulceration, hyperkeratosis)

Diagnosis

- history
- physical examination
- on the basis of major and minor criteria (Halliwell and Werner 1979)
  Major signs include:
- non-infective polyarthritis
- cutaneous lesions with supportive histopathological findings and positive immunofluorescence at the dermoepidermal junction
- Coombs'-positive anaemia
- Thrombocytopenia (platelet count below 50 000/mm^3) with or without a positive platelet function 3 test
- Glomerulonephritis with proteinuria
- Neutropenia
- Polymyositis
  Minor signs include:
- Fever
- Central nervous system signs, e.g. seizures, meningitis, polyneuropathy
- Pleuritis
  Definitive diagnosis of systemic lupus erythematosus requires the presence of two major signs or one major and two minor signs with supporting serological evidence.

SEROLOGICAL EVIDENCE

- positive antinuclear antibody test (ANA). Record the titre and compare with the normal for the laboratory performing the test
- positive lupus erythematosus cell preparation

CUTANEOUS BIOPSY

- inflammatory changes at the dermal—epidermal junctions; hydropic degeneration of the basal layer of the epidermis
- direct immunofluorescence reveals deposition of immunoglobulin or complement or both at the basement membrane zone

Differential diagnosis

- many dermatoses; systemic lupus erythematosus has been called the great imitator

Treatment

- glucocorticoids: prednisolone 2 mg/kg orally b.i.d.
- glucocorticoids and cytotoxic drugs: as described for pemphigus foliaceus
- other drugs which have been tried with varying benefit include: aspirin, chlorambucil orally at a dose of 0.2 mg/kg once daily, and levamisole at a dose of 2.5 mg/kg every 48 hours
- splenectomy (in some cases with severe haemolytic anaemia or thrombocytopenia)
- the prognosis is guarded although some dogs and cats may go into drug-free remission

IMMUNE-MEDIATED DISORDERS

Erythema multiforme

- dogs and cats
- rare
- the condition is an acute, but usually self-limiting eruption of the skin and/or mucous membranes

Causes

- there are many potential causes

DOGS
- folliculitis
- anal sacculitis
- drugs, e.g. aurothioglucose, antibacterial agents, thyroxine, levamisole, diethylcarbamazine
- idiopathic

CATS
- drugs, e.g. penicillin, aurothioglucose
- idiopathic

Clinical features

Variable:
- urticarial plaques
- vesicles, bullae and ulceration
- erythematous macules; these may spread out peripherally while healing at their centre
- some cases may be systemically ill

Diagnosis

- history
- physical examination
- biopsy findings vary according to the lesions

Differential diagnosis

- demodicosis
- folliculitis
- urticaria
- dermatophytosis
- autoimmune disorders

Treatment

- may spontaneously regress
- investigate and treat underlying cause if possible; remission is usually achieved by this means
- glucocorticoids are not usually beneficial

Toxic epidermal necrolysis

- dogs and cats
- rare
- causes include drugs (50% of cases), infections, malignancies, toxins and idiopathic

Clinical features

- any breed, sex or age
- acute onset with pyrexia, anorexia, lethargy and depression
- lesions may include: vesicles, bullae, ulceration, epidermal collarettes and skin necrosis
- lesion sites are most commonly the oral mucous membranes, mucocutaneous junctions and footpads
- the lesions are commonly painful and there may be a positive Nikolsky's sign

Diagnosis

- history
- physical examination
- biopsy: histological findings include hydropic degeneration of basal epidermal cells, dermoepidermal separation with subepidermal

vesicles, full-thickness epidermal necrosis with minimal dermal inflammation

Differential diagnosis

- pemphigus vulgaris
- bullous pemphigoid
- systemic lupus erythematosus
- erythema multiforme
- lymphoreticular neoplasia

Treatment

- correction of underlying cause
- symptomatic antibacterial and fluid therapy
- glucocorticoids are no longer favoured, most authorities now advising against their use
- prognosis guarded

Vasculitis

- rare
- dogs and cats
- associated with deposition of immune complex within blood-vessel wall, subsequent complement activation and chemotactic attraction of neutrophils
- causes include: bacteria, fungi, viruses, neoplasia, hypersensitivity to drugs and systemic lupus erythematosus. About 50% of cases are idiopathic, however

Clinical features

- cutaneous lesions are haemorrhagic bullae and ulcers, which tend to involve the extremities (paws, pinnae, tail)
- some cases are anorexic, febrile and depressed

Diagnosis

- history
- physical examination
- skin biopsy: neutrophilic, lymphocytic vasculitis

Differential diagnosis

- systemic lupus erythematosus

- cold agglutinin disease
- frost-bite, disseminated intravascular coagulation and lympho-reticular neoplasia

Treatment

- correction of underlying cause if possible
- immunosuppressive doses of glucocorticoids
- diaminodiphenylsulphone (dapsone, Ayerst) at 1 mg/kg t.i.d.

Linear immunoglobulin A dermatosis

- rare
- sterile pustular dermatosis recognized only in dachshunds of either sex
- biopsy shows intraepidermal pustular dermatitis with positive IgA immunofluorescence at the basement membrane zone
- treatment involves the use of immunosuppressive doses of glucocorticoids, or diaminodiphenylsulphone (dapsone, Ayerst) at a dose of 1 mg/kg t.i.d. orally

DISORDERS OF POSSIBLE IMMUNE MEDIATION

Cutaneous depigmentation and uveitis in dogs (Vogt–Koyanagi–Harada-like syndrome)

- dogs
- rare
- seen particularly in Akitas, Samoyeds and Siberian huskies
- no age or sex predilection

Clinical features

- simultaneous onset of anterior uveitis and depigmentation of the nose, eyelids and occasionally the footpads and anus
- photodermatitis may occur at depigmented sites

Diagnosis

- history
- physical examination
- skin biopsy: lichenoid interface dermatitis and marked pigmentary incontinence

Treatment

• for the treatment of anterior uveitis the reader is referred to ophthalmology textbooks. Accurate diagnosis and vigorous treatment is necessary to avoid possible blindness
• the cutaneous manifestations, if treated early, respond to glucocorticoids (prednisolone at a dose of 1 mg/kg s.i.d.) and thereafter on alternate days. Repigmentation may occur

Sterile eosinophilic pustulosis

• rare
• dogs
• any age, sex or breed

Clinical features

• acute onset
• lesions are pruritic, erythematous, annular, follicular and non-follicular, sterile, generalized pustules

Diagnosis

• history
• physical examination
• rule out other dermatoses
• haematology — eosinophilia
• biopsy: eosinophilic dermatitis and folliculitis

Differential diagnosis

• folliculitis
• dermatophyte infection
• pemphigus foliaceus
• subcorneal pustular dermatosis

Treatment

• immunosuppressive doses of glucocorticoids
• response is good although in most cases control but not cure is the rule

Sterile granuloma/pyogranuloma

• dogs principally — very rare in cats

- any age, sex or breed — with a predilection for the collie, Dobermann pinscher, Weimaraner, Great Dane, English bulldog, boxer and golden retriever

Clinical features

- lesions are papules, nodules or plaques
- sites affected include the head, pinnae or paws
- ulceration and secondary infection may occur

Diagnosis

- history
- physical examination
- biopsy: pyogranulomatous/granulomatous dermatitis

Differential diagnosis

- bacterial/mycotic/foreign-body granulomas
- neoplastic lesions

Treatment

- solitary lesions are excised
- for multiple lesions the treatment of choice is immunosuppressive doses of prednisolone. Remission is usually achieved within 7–10 days and maintained by alternate-day therapy

Alopecia areata

- rare
- dogs and cats
- may have an immune basis

Clinical features

- focal patches of non-inflammatory alopecia
- may occur anywhere — more commonly on the head, neck and trunk

Diagnosis

- history
- physical examination
- skin biopsy: the characteristic histopathological findings include a

peribulbar accumulation of lymphocytes, histiocytes and plasma cells

Differential diagnosis

- dermatophytosis
- demodicosis
- staphylococcal folliculitis
- endocrine disease

Treatment

- there is no effective treatment, some cases regress spontaneously. There is no clear evidence as to the efficacy of glucocorticoids

Feline plasma cell pododermatitis

- cats
- possibly immune-mediated

Clinical features

- soft, painless swelling of the footpads (Fig. 57)
- usually the central metacarpal or metatarsal pads
- occasionally one or more affected pads may ulcerate
- otherwise the cats are healthy
- a few cases have plasma cell stomatitis, with gingivitis and plaques at the palatine arches
- a few cases have glomerulonephritis or amyloidosis

Diagnosis

- history
- physical examination
- biopsy: superficial perivascular dermatitis/stomatitis with a predominance of plasma cells

Differential diagnosis

- other granulomatous lesions — infectious/sterile
- neoplastic lesions

Treatment

- no treatment is necessary in many cases

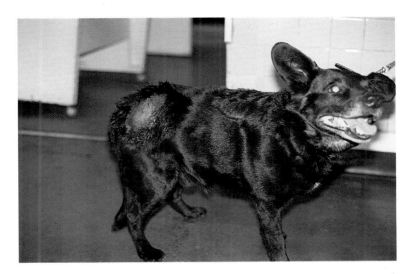

Fig. 1 Acute moist dermatitis on the gluteal region of a dog.

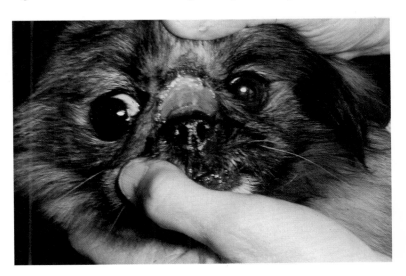

Fig. 2 Facial fold pyoderma in a Pekingese dog.

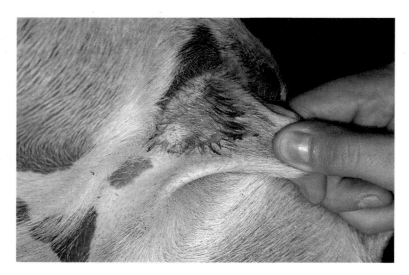

Fig. 3 Vulvar fold pyoderma in a bulldog.

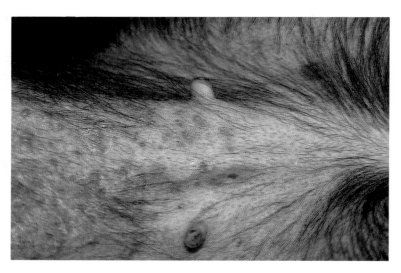

Fig. 4 Papules and pustules in the glabrous skin of the ventral abdomen of a dog with superficial pyoderma.

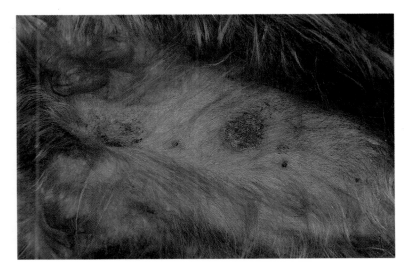

Fig. 5 Crusting lesion of superficial pyoderma in a dog.

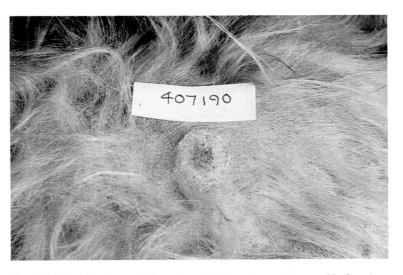

Fig. 6 Epidermal collarette lesion of superficial pyoderma (courtesy M. Geary).

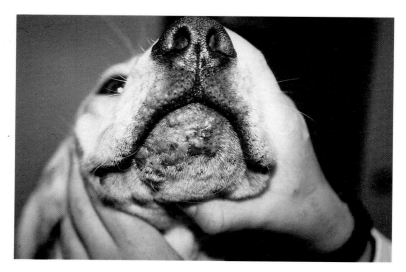

Fig. 7 Lesions of canine acne (courtesy I.S. Mason).

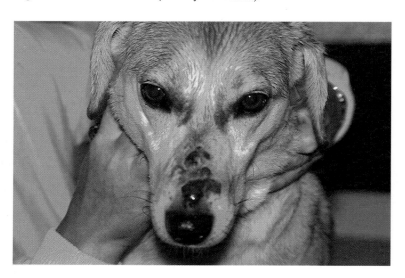

Fig. 8 Nasal pyoderma in a dog.

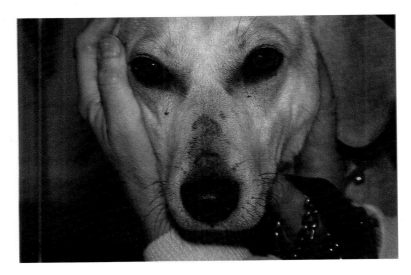

Fig. 9 Same dog as in Fig. 8 after treatment with potentiated sulphonamide for 3 weeks.

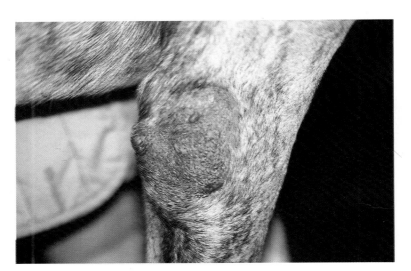

Fig. 10 Callus pyoderma on the elbow of a Great Dane.

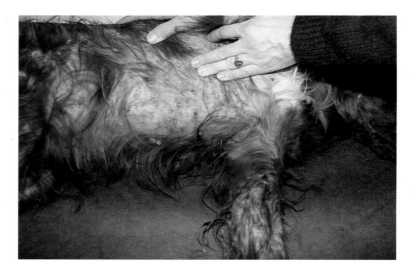

Fig. 11 Generalized deep pyoderma of the thorax and forelimb of an Irish setter.

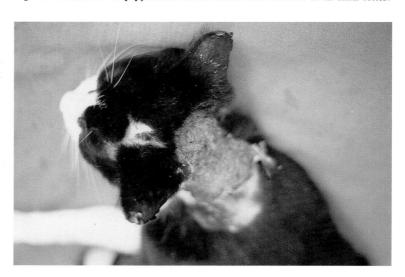

Fig. 12 Feline pyoderma in the neck region (cat-bite sepsis).

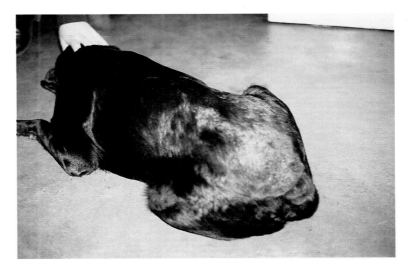

Fig. 13 Chronic flea-bite hypersensitivity in a Labrador dog.

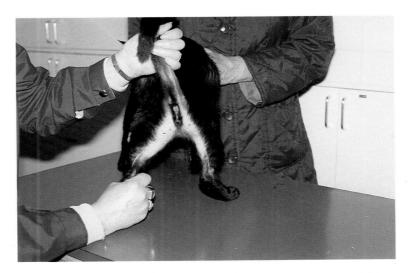

Fig. 14 Bilaterally symmetrical alopecia in a cat due to flea-bite hypersensitivity.

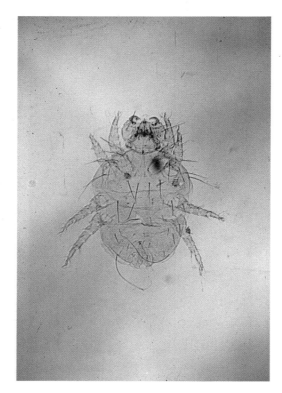

Fig. 15 *Cheyletiella* sp.
(courtesy M. Geary).

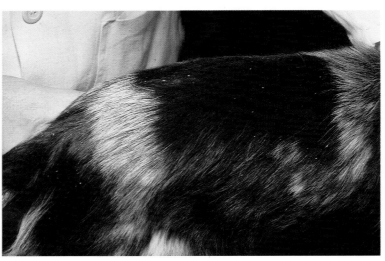

Fig. 16 Excessive scale in a spaniel due to *Cheyletiella* infestation.

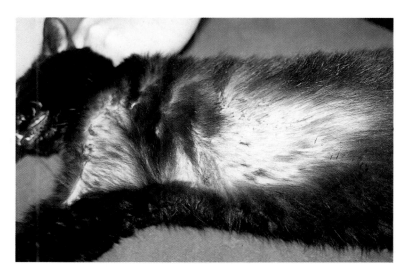

Fig. 17 Extensive alopecia and pruritic lesions in a cat with *Cheyletiella* infestation.

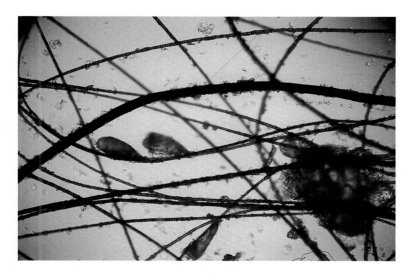

Fig. 18 *Cheyletiella* eggs attached to cat hairs (courtesy Mike Caygill).

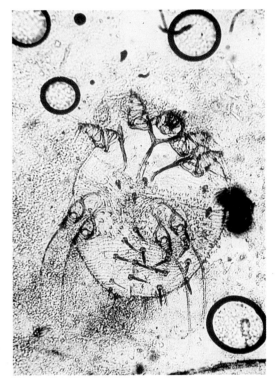

Fig. 19 *Sarcoptes scabiei* var. *canis*.

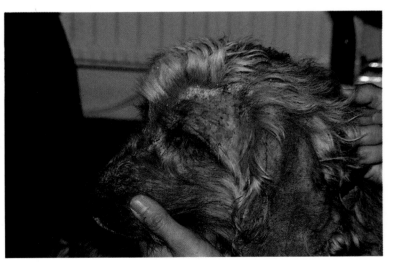

Fig. 20 Severe lesions of scabies in a cocker spaniel.

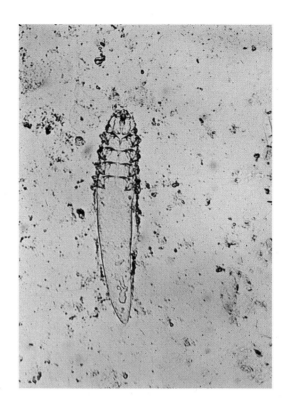

Fig. 21 *Demodex canis.*

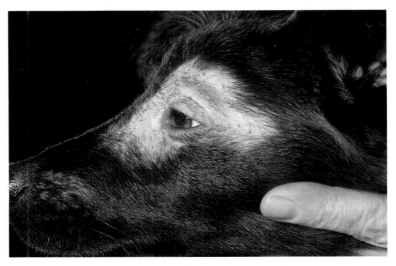

Fig. 22 Localized demodicosis in a dog.

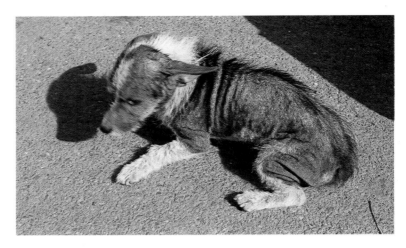

Fig. 23 Generalized squamous demodicosis in a Jack Russell terrier.

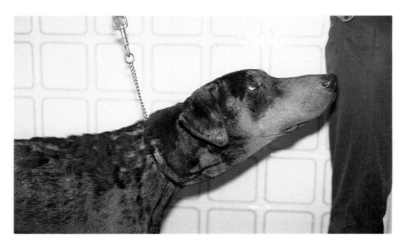

Fig. 24 Demodicosis in a 9-year-old Dobermann pinscher. The dog developed osteosarcoma of the ilium 2 months after onset of the demodicosis.

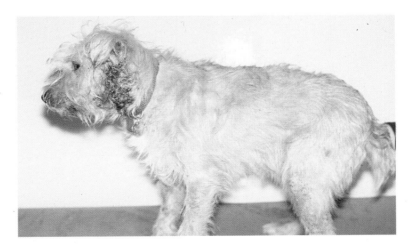

Fig. 25 Generalized demodicosis with secondary pyoderma in a 9-month-old crossbred dog.

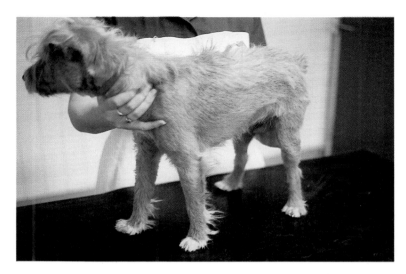

Fig. 26 Same dog as in Fig. 25 4 months after treatment with Amitraz and antibacterial agents.

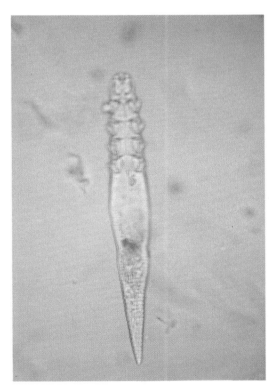

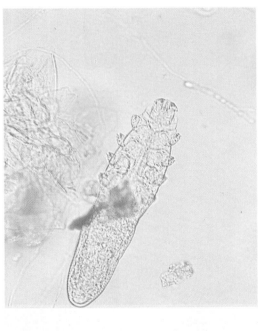

Fig. 27 *Demodex cati* (courtesy D. Scarff).

Fig. 28 Unnamed *Demodex* sp. of the cat (courtesy C. Chesney).

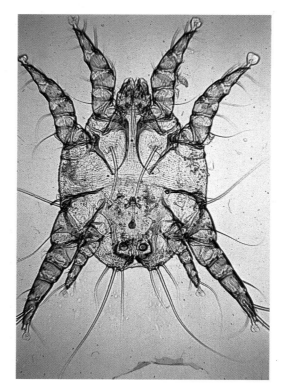

Fig. 29 *Otodectes cynotis.*

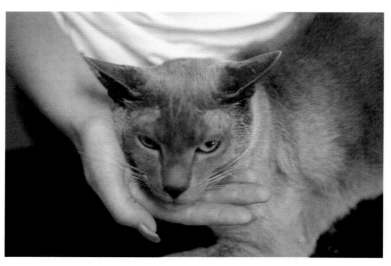

Fig. 30 Erythematous facial lesions in a cat due to hypersensitivity to *Otodectes*.

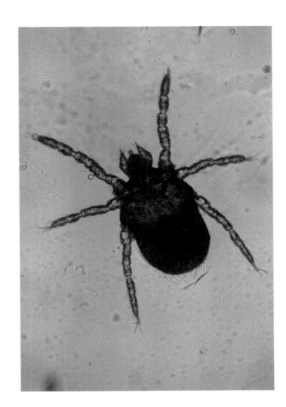

Fig. 31 *Neotrombicula autumnalis* (courtesy L.R. Thomsett).

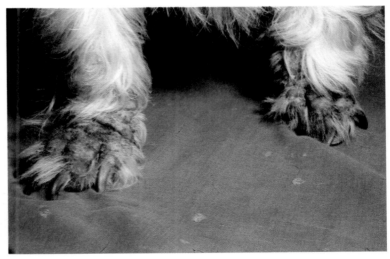

Fig. 32 Pododermatitis in a West Highland white terrier due to hypersensitivity to *Neotrombicula autumnalis* (courtesy K.L. Thoday).

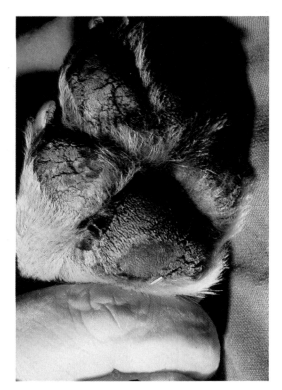

Fig. 33 Ulceration and hyperkeratosis of the footpads of a dog due to hookworm larvae (courtesy K.L. Thoday).

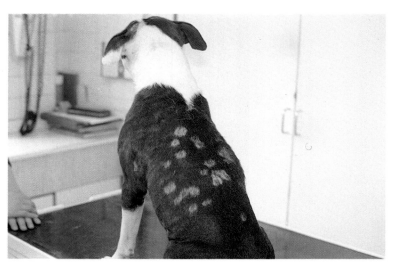

Fig. 34 Generalized circular lesions of *Microsporum canis* in a dog.

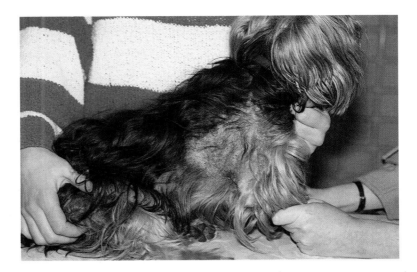

Fig. 35 Alopecia on the thorax of a Yorkshire terrier due to *Trichophyton mentagrophytes*.

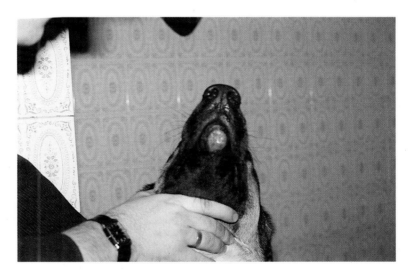

Fig. 36 Kerion lesion due to *Microsporum canis* on the chin of a German shepherd dog.

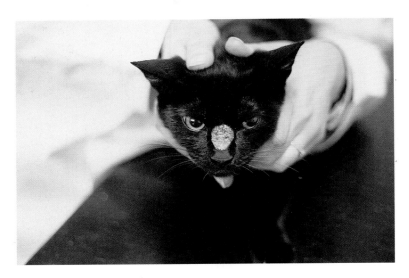

Fig. 37 *Microsporum canis* lesion in a cat.

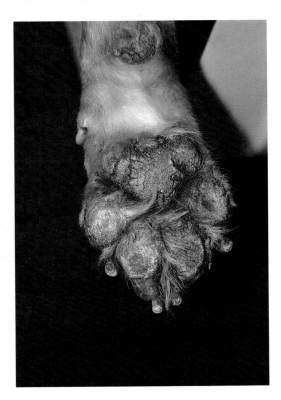

Fig. 38 Hyperkeratosis of the footpads of a dog with distemper virus infection.

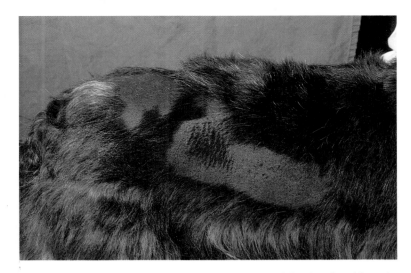

Fig. 39 Bilaterally symmetrical alopecia due to hypothyroidism in a Scottish terrier.

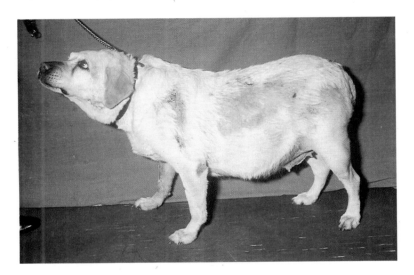

Fig. 40 Pendulous abdomen in a yellow Labrador with hyperadrenocorticism (courtesy K.L. Thoday).

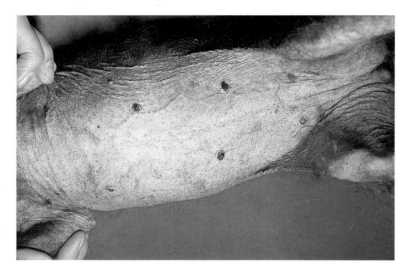

Fig. 41 Thin inelastic skin of the ventral abdomen of a miniature poodle with hyperadrenocorticism (courtesy K.L. Thoday).

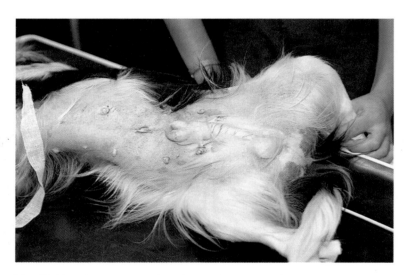

Fig. 42 Alopecia, gynaecomastia and pendulous prepuce in a King Charles spaniel with Sertoli's cell tumour.

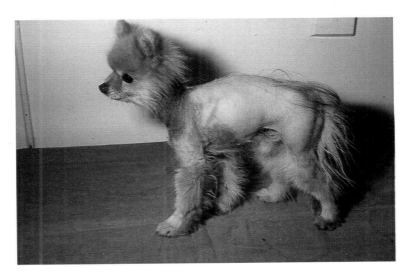

Fig. 43 Growth hormone-responsive alopecia in a 2-year-old male Pomeranian (courtesy K.L. Thoday).

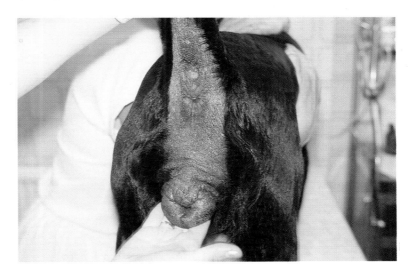

Fig. 44 Alopecia, hyperpigmentation and lichenification in an 8-year-old Labrador with hyperoestrogenism. Note the enlarged vulva. There was a granulosa cell tumour of the ovary.

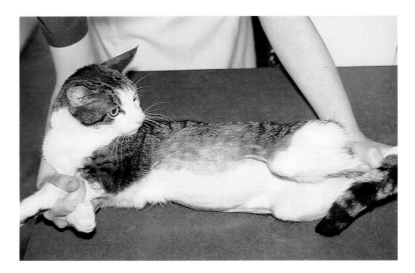

Fig. 45 Feline symmetric alopecia affecting the trunk.

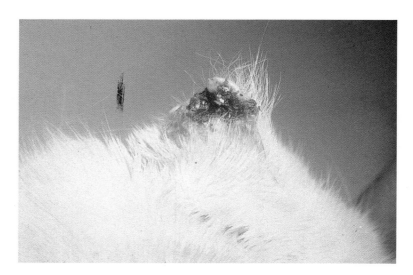

Fig. 46 Squamous cell carcinoma of the tip of the pinna in a cat.

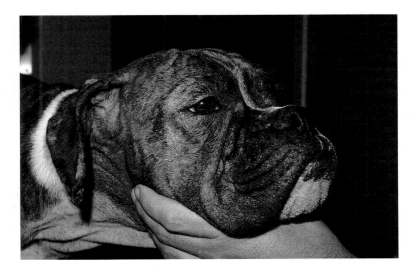

Fig. 47 Periocular alopecia and erythema in a boxer with atopy.

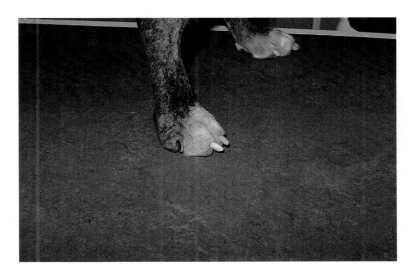

Fig. 48 Pedal erythema in the same dog as in Fig. 47.

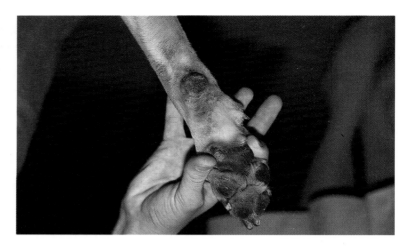

Fig. 49 Erythema and alopecia below the stop pad of a yellow Labrador with atopy.

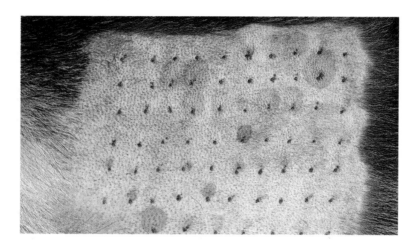

Fig. 50 Positive intradermal allergy test in a German shepherd dog (courtesy Dr I.S. Mason).

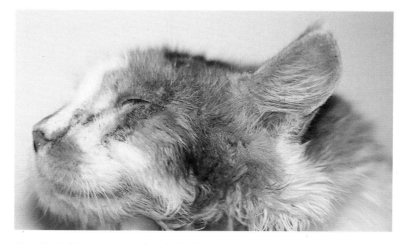

Fig. 51 Facial erythema and periorbital scabs in a cat with milk hypersensitivity.

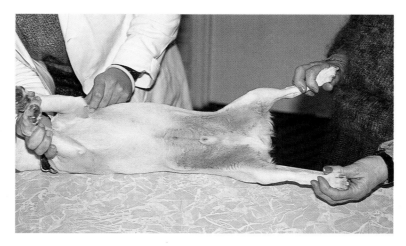

Fig. 52 Acute erythema of the glabrous skin of the ventral abdomen of a dog with contact hypersensitivity to grass pollen.

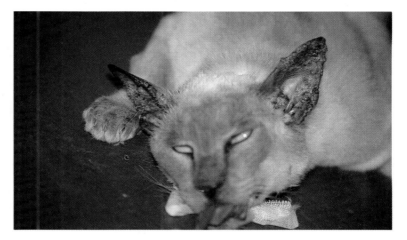

Fig. 53 Severe crusting of the ears of a cat with pemphigus foliaceus.

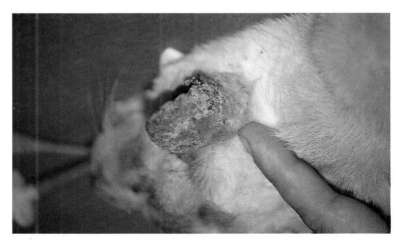

Fig. 54 Close-up of the pinna of the same cat as in Fig. 53.

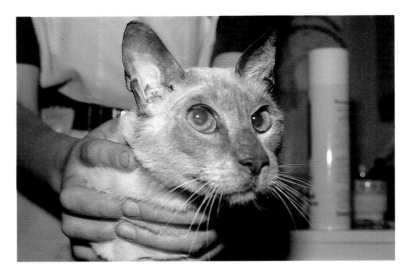

Fig. 55 Same cat as in Figs. 53 and 54 following glucocorticoids and chrysotherapy.

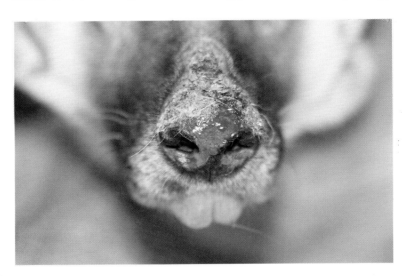

Fig. 56 Nasal lesion of discoid lupus erythematosus.

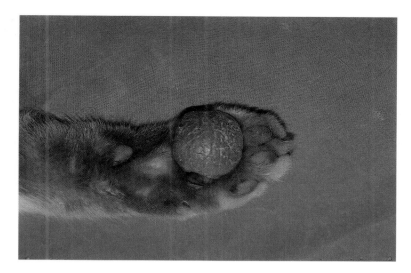

Fig. 57 Plasma cell pododermatitis affecting the central metacarpal pad of a cat.

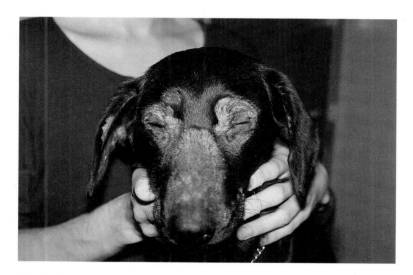

Fig. 58 Facial crusting lesions in a dog with zinc-responsive dermatosis.

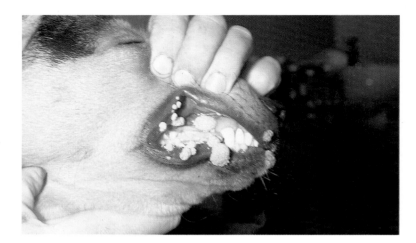

Fig. 59 Canine oral papillomata.

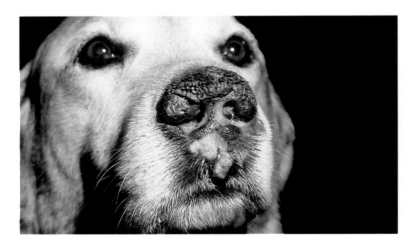

Fig. 60 Squamous cell carcinoma affecting the nose of a dog (courtesy K.L. Thoday).

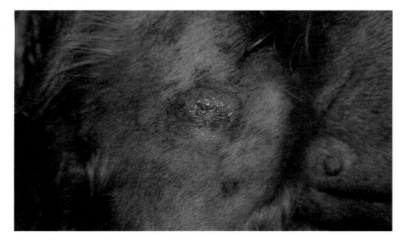

Fig. 61 Solitary mast cell tumour affecting the hind limb of a dog.

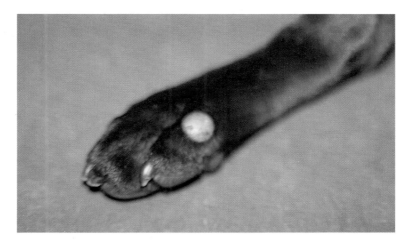

Fig. 62 Histiocytoma affecting the foot of a dog.

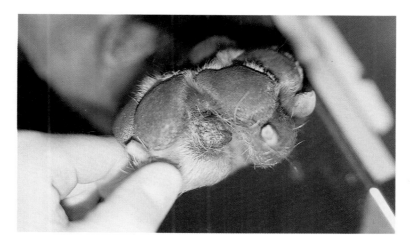

Fig. 63 Interdigital melanoma in a dog.

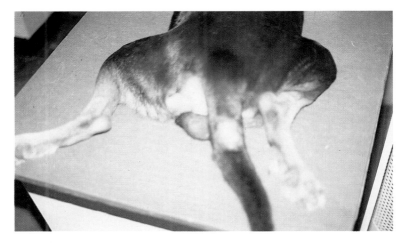

Fig. 64 Tail gland hyperplasia in a dog with a testicular tumour.

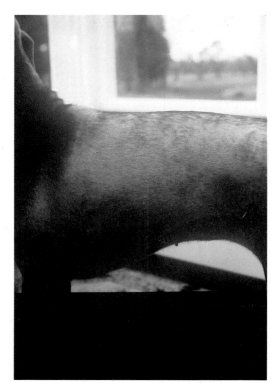

Fig. 65 Colour mutant alopecia in a 3-year-old Dobermann pinscher.

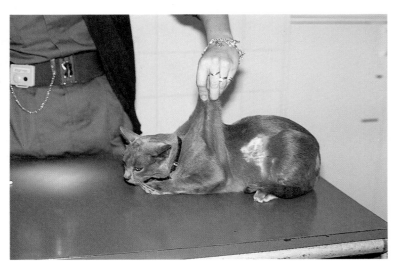

Fig. 66 Extreme skin extensibility in a cat with cutaneous asthenia.

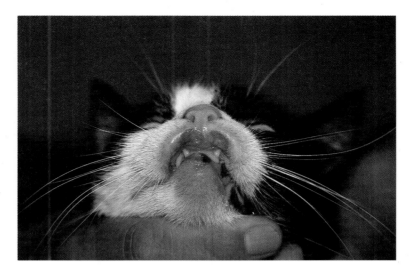

Fig. 67 Indolent ulcer in a cat.

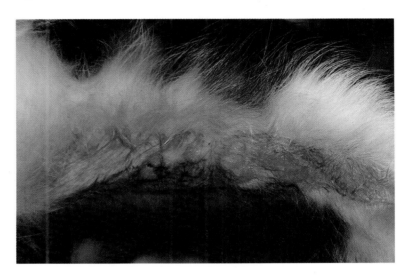

Fig. 68 Eosinophilic plaque lesions on the abdomen of a cat.

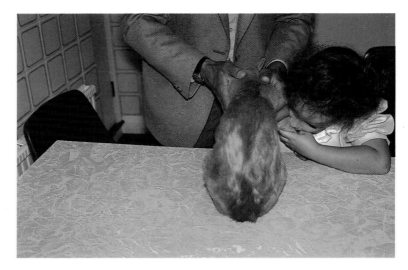

Fig. 69 Psychogenic alopecia affecting the dorsum of a Siamese cat.

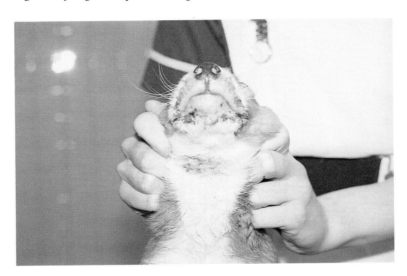

Fig. 70 Juvenile cellulitis. Crusting around the lips and marked submandibular lymphadenopathy.

- supportive treatment for ulcerative lesions
- immunosuppressive doses of glucocorticoids
- chrysotherapy as for pemphigus foliaceus

Feline hypereosinophilic syndrome

- cats
- rare
- possibly immune-mediated
- no age, sex or breed predilection

Clinical features

- many organs may be infiltrated by eosinophils, e.g. spleen, liver, bone marrow and lymph nodes
- this infiltration results in multisystem organ dysfunction
- occasionally there is infiltration of the skin by eosinophils, resulting in a severely pruritic, erythematous dermatosis

Diagnosis

- history
- physical examination
- haematology
- biopsy: histopathological findings include a superficial and deep perivascular dermatitis with a predominance of eosinophils

Differential diagnosis

- this is lengthy and depends on which organs are involved

Treatment

- there is no effective treatment
- the prognosis is poor

9/Nutritional Skin Disease

GENERAL POINTS

- in healthy dogs and cats fed on reputable canned pet foods nutritional deficiencies or imbalances are highly unlikely
- animals fed entirely on generic foods or dried food may develop scaling, crusting dermatoses; in such animals intensive investigation of their dermatological problem may fail to identify the cause, but a significant improvement is seen on feeding well-balanced diets
- in all cases suspected of having a nutritional basis, therefore, a careful history and assessment of the suitability of the diet is necessary
- important skin diseases which respond to dietary supplementation include:

  protein deficiency
  essential fatty acid deficiency
  vitamin deficiency — notably A, B and E
  zinc deficiency (zinc-responsive dermatosis)

PROTEIN DEFICIENCY

- the diet should consist of at least 25% protein on a dry-matter basis as a percentage of calorific intake
- protein deficiency may arise as a result of starvation, feeding an incorrect diet too low in protein, maldigestion, malabsorption, or excessive protein loss from the gut (protein-losing enteropathy) or from the kidneys (nephrotic syndrome)

Clinical features

- the coat is thin, poor and with thin brittle hairs that easily fall out, leading to patchy alopecia
- there may be generalized, crusting lesions over most of the body
- there may also be epidermal hyperpigmentation, with loss of hair pigment
- lesions tend to be more severe in young dogs due to their increased protein requirement

Diagnosis

- history, e.g. known history of starvation, feeding home-prepared diet inadequate in protein

- physical examination
- investigation of possible systemic diseases listed above

Treatment

- feed a diet that has adequate protein
- treat any systemic disease

ESSENTIAL FATTY ACID DEFICIENCY

- dogs and cats
- may be seen in animals fed on dry diets to the exclusion of everything else, home-prepared diets too low in fat, or commercial diets that have been stored incorrectly allowing fat to become rancid
- may also be seen in association with pancreatic disease, hepatic disease and intestinal malabsorption
- dog food requires 3% of fat in a canned diet and 8% in a dry diet; the requirement for cats is much higher since $35-40\%$ of their calorific intake is normally provided by fats
- cats lack the ability to convert linolenic and linoleic acid to arachidonic acid due to a deficiency of the enzyme δ-6-desaturase; there is therefore a necessity for animal fat in the cat's diet, or a deficiency of arachidonic acid results

Clinical features

- several months on a deficient diet are necessary prior to the development of lesions
- poor, lack-lustre coat
- initially a scaliness of the skin with patchy alopecia, later seborrhoea oleosa, secondary pyoderma and acanthosis
- sebum is initially decreased in quantity and later increases, accounting for the initial scaliness with subsequent seborrhoea oleosa

Diagnosis

- history
- physical examination
- biopsy: there may be abnormal keratinization with epidermal hyperplasia, hypergranulosis and orthokeratotic hyperplasia
- response to treatment

Treatment

- feed a nutritionally adequate diet
- treat any underlying systemic disease
- supplement the diet with one teaspoonful of equal parts of vegetable oil and animal fat or Efavet capsules (Efamol, UK)
- response usually occurs within 1–3 months

VITAMIN IMBALANCES

Vitamin A

- vitamin A is present in fish oils and in liver and kidney
- it is extremely efficiently stored in the liver, and deficiency is highly unlikely in clinical practice in animals fed on commercial diets
- a vitamin A-responsive dermatosis was first described in two cocker spaniels and a miniature schnauzer (Ihrke and Goldschmidt 1983) and there have been a number of similar reports since then
- the cases are not associated with an absolute deficiency of vitamin A. Therapeutic success may be due to an excess of the vitamin A either meeting the need brought about by localized deficiency or overriding a partial metabolic impairment of its utilization

Clinical features

- generalized seborrhoea initially, with later seborrhoeic dermatitis and the development of tenacious frond-like keratinous plugs, especially on the ventral chest and abdomen

Diagnosis

- history
- physical examination
- investigation of other possible causes of seborrhoea
- biopsy: extreme follicular hyperplasia with minimal surface hyperkeratosis
- response to therapy

Treatment

- 10 000 units of vitamin A orally per day
- response generally occurs within 3 weeks
- treatment needs to be continued for life

Vitamin B

- deficiencies of vitamin B complex are extremely unlikely in practice

Biotin deficiency

- has been produced experimentally in dogs and cats
- deficiency may also result from prolonged antibacterial therapy, or by feeding a diet which is high in uncooked eggs (egg white contains avidin, which interferes with the absorption of biotin)

Clinical features

- in dogs there may be periorbital alopecia in mild cases, with generalized crusting lesions, lethargy, emaciation and diarrhoea in severe cases
- in cats miliary dermatitis has been reported anecdotally (see pp. 166−167)

Niacin deficiency

- has been produced by diets low in animal protein and high in cereals. Cereals have low levels of tryptophan, which is converted by dogs (not cats) to niacin

Clinical features

- pruritus and dermatitis of the legs and abdomen
- ulcerated mucous membranes
- diarrhoea and emaciation

Riboflavin deficiency

- if there is any meat or dairy product in the diet this deficiency is virtually impossible

Clinical features

- experimental cases or dogs and cats on a grossly deficient diet exhibit seborrhoea sicca as the prominent sign, with alopecia of the head in the cat

Treatment of vitamin B deficiency

- brewer's yeast or injections of vitamin B complex

Vitamin E

- naturally occurring vitamin E deficiency has not been reported in the dog
- in cats may result from excessive fat in the diet, such as exclusive feeding of canned red tuna fish, or from oxidation of fat during prolonged storage
- in experimental dogs vitamin E deficiency results in severe suppression of *in vitro* lymphocyte blastogenesis
- cats develop pansteatitis

Clinical features

DOGS • generalized erythematous seborrhoea sicca with a tendency to develop secondary pyoderma

CATS • affected cats are anorexic, resent palpation and may become excitable when handled
- the subcutaneous tissue, and sometimes abdominal fat, is firm and lumpy on palpation

Diagnosis

- history
- physical examination
- biopsy: in dogs the histopathological findings are non-specific, consisting of hyperplastic superficial perivascular dermatitis. In cats there is a lobular panniculitis; ceroid, a pink homogeneous material when stained with H and E, is found in lipocytes, giant cells and macrophages

Treatment

- vitamin E at a dose of 13.5 IU/kg daily
- in cats this treatment will need to be supplemented with systemic glucocorticoids in order to reduce inflammation and pain
- vitamin E at a dose of 400 to 800 IU b.i.d. has been used to treat certain autoimmune disorders such as discoid lupus erythematosus, suggesting an immunosuppressive effect

ZINC-RESPONSIVE DERMATOSIS

- most cases have been reported in dogs
- in kittens a dietary deficiency of zinc has been shown to cause a thin poor coat, with scaliness of the skin and ulceration of the buccal margins

• in the UK virtually all cases reported in dogs have resulted from the feeding of soya- and/or cereal-based diets, possibly in some dogs in association with an inherent defect of zinc absorption
• dry diets contain high levels of phytate and calcium, which bind zinc, rendering it less available for absorption
• over-supplementation of a growing dog with calcium may produce similar symptoms

Clinical signs

• any breed, age or sex. Alaskan malamutes, Siberian huskies, Dobermanns and Great Danes may be predisposed
• although two different types were originally described (Kunkle 1980), there is considerable overlap between the two
• signs include a harsh coat, crusting lesions of the head, limbs, scrotum and perineum (Fig. 58)
• also noted is seborrhoea sicca, ceruminous otitis and peripheral lymphadenopathy

Diagnosis

• history
• physical examination
• laboratory tests — plasma zinc measurement, special plastic and low-metal tubes (Becton Dickinson) are required
• skin biopsy (Thoday 1989): parakeratosis — not all cases, however
• response to therapy — in practice the most useful test

Treatment

• oral zinc sulphate capsules (Zincomed, Medo Pharmaceuticals) at a dose of 10 mg/kg/day
• to reduce the risk of gastric irritation and vomiting, the drug is given with food
• most cases show a good response within 3 weeks
• the diet is then changed to canned meat and biscuits, which obviates the need to continue with zinc supplementation
• rarely, in cases of genetic defects of zinc absorption in some malamutes, zinc supplementation may be required for life
• most dry diets now have added zinc and the condition is therefore less common

10/Neoplastic Skin Disease

GENERAL POINTS

- cutaneous neoplasms are common, representing approximately 30% of all canine tumours and 20% of all feline tumours
- usually older animals are affected but in some tumours, for example, histiocytoma and papilloma, occurrence is in younger animals
- the boxer, basset-hound, Weimaraner, Kerry blue terrier, Norwegian elkhound and Scottish terrier are in general predisposed to cutaneous neoplasms
- there is no breed predisposition in the cat
- feline skin tumours are more commonly malignant than canine cases
- in the majority of cases specific diagnosis can *only* be made by biopsy and histopathological examination
- in this text details of treatment and histopathology are not discussed; but further information can be found in the 'Selected Reading' section, pp. 183–184

CLASSIFICATION OF SKIN TUMOURS

- epithelial neoplasms
- mesenchymal neoplasms
- lymphohistiocytic neoplasms
- melanocytic neoplasms
- secondary cutaneous neoplasms
- non-neoplastic tumours

EPITHELIAL NEOPLASMS

Papilloma (wart)

DOGS
- benign
- common
- in the young dog they tend to occur around the lips and in the oral cavity (Fig. 59); this type is contagious and caused by deoxyribonucleic acid (DNA) papovavirus with an incubation period of approximately 30 days
- in older dogs of 8 to 10 years or more, solitary papillomas are

very common and can occur anywhere on the body, but particularly the head and feet
- the oral form may cause problems with eating and may haemorrhage; in older dogs papillomas are insignificant unless trauma causes haemorrhage or the owner considers them to be unsightly

CATS
- rare
- older cats
- benign

Treatment

- surgical excision or cryosurgery
- the viral form in young dogs usually undergoes spontaneous regression within 3 months; only if there is interference with eating is surgery indicated
- autogenous wart vaccines may be tried but their usefulness is debatable
- advise the owners of older dogs prior to surgery that new warts may develop at a later stage

Intracutaneous cornifying epithelioma (keratoacanthoma)

- dogs
- uncommon
- benign
- mainly young dogs, less than 5 years of age, and more commonly male
- Norwegian elkhounds and keeshonds are predisposed to the multiple form
- tumours are usually solitary, except in the breeds mentioned above, and tend to occur on the back, neck, thorax and shoulders
- they vary from 1 to 4 cm in diameter, and have a central pore, which may have a keratin plug, opening to the surface of the skin

Treatment

- surgical excision
- the multiple form may cause problems since new tumours tend to develop after surgical excision

Squamous cell carcinoma

- common, malignant tumour arising from the squamous epithelial cells

DOGS
- any breed, but Scottish terriers, Pekingese, boxer, poodle and Norwegian elkhound may be predisposed
- usually older dogs (9 years or more)
- common sites include the digits, lips and external nares (Fig. 60)
- the tumours are usually solitary, hairless and tend to ulcerate
- local invasion is common and metastasis to the regional lymph nodes and lungs may occur
- squamous cell carcinoma of the digits carries a particularly guarded prognosis

CATS
- older cats
- white cats or cats with white ears are particularly predisposed
- the most common sites are the pinna, nose, lips and eyelids (Fig. 46)

Treatment

- surgical excision; particularly effective for pinna squamous cell carcinoma, with good cosmetic results
- cryosurgery
- radiotherapy

Basal cell tumour

- benign
- dogs and cats, but more commonly in cats
- usually older animals
- in dogs, cocker spaniels, poodles and Kerry blues are predisposed
- the tumour is usually solitary, firm and rounded, up to several centimetres in diameter
- tend to occur on the head and neck
- ulceration and alopecia over the surface is common

Treatment

- none
- surgical excision or cryosurgery

HAIR FOLLICLE TUMOURS

Trichoepithelioma

DOGS
- benign
- common

- cocker spaniel and basset-hound predisposed
- tends to occur on the back and shoulders
- usually solitary, round and well circumscribed, and between 0.5 and 10 cm in diameter
- growth is slow, local invasion is very rare
- the tumour may ulcerate

CATS
- rare
- more likely to occur on the head

Treatment

- none
- surgical excision

Pilomatrixoma

- thought to arise from the hair matrix
- uncommon in the dog, extremely rare in the cat
- most commonly seen in the poodle and the Kerry blue
- usually occurs on the back
- metastasis to the lungs occurs very rarely

Tricholemmoma

- uncommon
- dogs, 5 to 13 years of age
- benign neoplasm that arises from the outer root sheath of hair follicles
- firm, rounded up to 7 cm in diameter
- occur most commonly on the head and neck

Dilated pore of Winer

- benign
- cats, older males predisposed
- solitary
- occur on the face and neck
- smooth cyst-like structure with a central keratin-filled pore

Treatment

- none
- surgical excision

SEBACEOUS GLAND TUMOURS

These tumours are either adenomas, epitheliomas or adeno-carcinomas.
- common in older dogs
- cocker spaniel, Kerry blue, Boston terrier, beagle, dachshund and basset-hound are predisposed
- tumours develop anywhere on the body

Adenomas

- usually slow-growing, multiple
- 0.5−2 cm in diameter
- may haemorrhage if traumatized

Epitheliomas

- similar to basal cell tumours in appearance

Adenocarcinomas

- distinguished from adenomas by rapid growth
- tend to be larger — more than 2 cm in diameter
- metastasis is rare

Treatment

- none
- surgical resection
- cryosurgery

SWEAT GLAND TUMOURS

- uncommon
- dogs and cats
- most arise from the epitrichial (apocrine) glands

Epitrichial adenomas

- older dogs and cats
- single, well-circumscribed and slow-growing

Epitrichial adenocarcinomas

- these are rapidly invasive and metastasis is common

Atrichial (eccrine) adenomas and adenocarcinomas

- arise from the eccrine sweat glands of the footpads
- dogs and cats
- extremely rare

Treatment

- leave
- surgical excision or cryosurgery

PERIANAL GLAND TUMOURS

Perianal adenomas

- common
- dogs — usually males, rare in females
- the majority arise from the circumanal glands of the perianal area
- occasionally occur on the ventral part of the tail, prepuce and lumbosacral area
- cocker spaniels, beagles, English bulldogs, Afghans, dachshunds and Samoyeds are predisposed
- slow-growing, firm, nodular tumours with a high tendency to ulcerate and bleed; anal irritation is a frequent finding

Treatment

- castration is the treatment of choice as 95% of these tumours will respond
- ulcerated tumours will need surgical removal
- prior to surgery it is useful to administer 5−10 mg of oestradiol benzoate (Intervet) weekly by subcutaneous injection for a few weeks in order to reduce the size of the tumour. Prolonged administration of oestrogens is not indicated due to the risk of bone marrow suppression
- castration is performed concurrently with the surgical removal of the tumour

Perianal adenocarcinomas

- rare
- occur in equal frequency in males and females
- rapidly growing malignant tumour
- widespread metastasis is common

Treatment

- surgical excision is difficult, may metastasize or recur locally
- cryosurgery
- radiotherapy
- oestrogen therapy or castration is *not* effective

MESENCHYMAL NEOPLASMS

Fibroma

- dogs and cats
- no breed predisposition in cats; breeds of dogs predisposed include boxers, Boston terriers and fox-terriers
- more common in female dogs
- may occur anywhere on the body — more commonly on the limbs, flank and groin

Treatment

- surgical excision
- none

Fibrovascular papilloma

- dogs
- common
- benign
- large and giant breeds are predisposed
- the tumour may be solitary or multiple, and is usually small (< 1 cm long)
- the most frequent sites are the ventral thorax and the extremities

Treatment

- surgical excision or cryosurgery
- leave

Fibrosarcoma

- dogs and cats
- common
- malignant

DOGS   • older dogs

- the cocker spaniel and females are predisposed
- the tumour is often solitary with a predilection for the limbs and trunk
- growth is rapid and infiltrative, but metastasis occurs in less than 25% of cases

CATS
- seen in kittens and older cats
- in kittens less than 4 months of age, the tumour has been shown to be caused by feline sarcoma virus, a mutant of feline leukaemia virus; such kittens have positive titres to feline leukaemia virus and in these cases the tumour is multicentric
- in older cats the tumours are not induced by feline sarcoma virus
- predilection sites in older cats are the limbs, trunk and head

Treatment

- wide surgical excision
- local recurrence occurs in about 30% of dogs
- the most useful prognostic sign in dogs and cats is the mitotic index
- radiotherapy and chemotherapy are of limited benefit once metastasis has occurred

Lipoma

- dogs and cats
- older animals ($>$ 8 years)
- common in dogs, rare in cats
- benign tumour of subcutaneous lipocytes
- cocker spaniels, dachshunds, Weimaraners, Labrador retrievers, terriers and obese females are predisposed
- well-circumscribed, soft, subcutaneous swellings, 1–30 cm in diameter, which are most commonly found on the trunk and abdomen

Treatment

- surgical excision
- none
- does not recur or metastasize

Liposarcoma

- rare
- dogs and cats

- malignant tumour arising from dermal or subcutaneous fibroblasts
- older dogs, male dachshunds and Brittany spaniels are predisposed
- usually solitary; typical sites are the ventral abdomen and thorax
- metastasis is uncommon

Treatment

- wide, early surgical excision

TUMOURS OF VASCULAR ORIGIN

Haemangioma

- uncommon in dogs and rare in cats
- benign neoplasm arising from the endothelial cells of blood-vessels
- boxers may be predisposed
- older dogs and cats
- usually a solitary tumour, which occurs on the flank, limbs and head; slow-growing, firm, well-circumscribed, 0.5 − 3 cm in diameter

Treatment

- surgical excision; haemorrhage may be a problem

Haemangiosarcoma

- dogs and cats
- uncommon
- malignant tumour arising from the endothelial cells of blood-vessels
- German shepherd dogs, boxers and Bernese mountain dogs are predisposed
- the tumour is usually solitary, rapidly growing and invasive; ulceration is common

Treatment

- wide surgical excision
- recurrence is common
- there is early metastasis in the dog, in cats metastasis is less common; in both cats and dogs, however, the prognosis is poor, especially in dogs, with a mean survival time of 4 months following diagnosis, response to radiotherapy and chemotherapy being poor

Haemangiopericytoma

- mainly dogs, extremely rare in the cat
- older animals
- German shepherd dog, boxer, springer and cocker spaniel, and fox-terrier are predisposed
- the tumour is solitary, firm, large (2–25 cm in diameter), well circumscribed and usually occurs on the limbs
- metastasis is rare

Treatment

- radical surgical excision
- recurrence is common and sometimes amputation of the affected limb is necessary

TUMOURS OF NEURAL ORIGIN

Perineural fibroblastoma (Schwannoma)

- rare
- dogs and cats
- arise from the nerve sheath (Schwann cells)

DOGS
- most are benign
- usually solitary, firm, subcutaneous swellings on limbs
- there may be nerve dysfunction in some cases

CATS
- most are malignant
- occur anywhere on the body
- clinically similar in appearance to the tumour in the dog

Treatment

DOGS
- surgical resection; even with benign forms local recurrence is common

CATS
- surgical excision; local recurrence is likely, metastasis is common
- radiotherapy and chemotherapy are of minimal benefit

Mast cell tumour (mastocytoma, mastocytosis)

- dogs and cats
- common neoplasms of mast cells
- benign or malignant

DOGS
- breeds predisposed include boxers, Boston terriers, bulldogs, Labrador retrievers, Staffordshire bull-terriers and Weimaraners
- any age but more common in the older dog
- usually solitary (occasionally multiple) dermal or subcutaneous tumours, 1–10 cm in diameter, which arise most frequently on the perineum, hind limbs (Fig. 61) and trunk
- malignant mastocytomas (approximately 30% of the total) extend into the subcutaneous tissue, are ulcerative and spread to the regional lymph nodes. Tumours located on the scrotum, prepuce and perineal region are often highly malignant
- some mast cell tumours release histamine, heparin and other vasoactive amines. This may lead to severe inflammation and pruritus at the tumour site, and, systemically, gastric ulceration, duodenal ulceration, bleeding disorders, defective antibody synthesis and glomerulitis

CATS
- usually multiple tumours
- the majority are malignant
- no breed incidence
- firm, nodular swellings 0.5–5 cm in diameter, which commonly arise on the head
- systemic complications may occur as in the dog
- metastasis occurs early and the prognosis is very poor

Diagnosis

- history
- physical examination
- biopsy

Treatment

- for solitary tumours use wide surgical excision
- other treatment regimes depend on the clinical stage of the tumour, and may involve radiation therapy, systemic glucocorticoids, cimetidine (Tagamet, Smith Klyne and French) and intralesional steroids. Details of clinical staging and treatment have been described (Tams and Macy 1981)

LYMPHOHISTIOCYTIC NEOPLASMS

Histiocytoma

- dogs, extremely rare in the cat
- common tumour arising from the histiocytes

- breeds predisposed include the boxer, Labrador retriever, Great Dane and cocker spaniel
- usually solitary; common sites are the head, neck, trunk and feet (Fig. 62)
- the tumour is rapidly growing, up to 2 cm in diameter
- alopecia and erythema are common on the surface
- histologically these tumours have numerous mitotic figures suggesting to a non-veterinary pathologist a high degree of malignancy; however, histiocytomas are always benign and never metastasize

Treatment

- surgical excision is curative; most tumours regress spontaneously within 3 months, so it is not necessary to perform surgery on asymptomatic tumours

Fibrous histiocytoma

- rare
- dogs and cats (extremely rare)
- younger dogs 2−4 years of age; collies seem to be predisposed
- generally multiple, firm, well-circumscribed, nodular tumours 0.5−7 cm in diameter
- common sites are the face and feet; the tumour may also occur on the cornea

Treatment

- surgical excision
- sublesional injection of 10−40 mg of methylprednisolone (Depomedrone V, Upjohn)

Malignant fibrous histiocytoma

- rare
- older dogs and cats
- malignant
- solitary, firm, invasive tumours, which tend to occur on the limbs and neck

Treatment

- wide surgical excision; metastasis occurs late in the course of the disease

Transmissible venereal tumour

- uncommon
- dogs
- tumour cells contain 59 chromosomes (normal canine cells have 78)
- cause unknown; possibly viral
- transmission usually by coitus, but also by licking, biting and scratching

Clinical features

- dogs of any age, sex or breed; young dogs particularly
- neoplastic lesions may be multiple or single, pedunculated, firm or friable, 1–20 cm in diameter; ulceration is frequent
- common sites are the penis and vagina, and the skin of the face and limbs
- in experimental dogs the tumour has been found to be benign, and in many cases regresses spontaneously; in naturally occurring cases, however, metastasis is frequent, and the incidence of spontaneous remission is unknown, so treatment is always indicated

Diagnosis

- history
- physical examination
- biopsy

Treatment

- surgical excision
- radiotherapy
- combination chemotherapy: vincristine 0.0125–0.025 mg/kg intravenously weekly; cyclophosphamide 1 mg/kg orally; methotrexate 0.3–0.5 mg/kg weekly
- single-agent chemotherapy: vincristine 0.025 mg/kg intravenously weekly

Cutaneous lymphosarcoma

- rare
- dogs and cats
- in cats caused usually by feline leukaemia virus (FeLV)
- there are two forms: primary cutaneous lymphosarcoma, originating in the skin, and a secondary form arising from dissemination from lymphosarcoma at another site

- mostly older animals are affected, although the tumour can occur at any age

Primary cutaneous lymphosarcoma

- histologically primary cutaneous lymphosarcoma may be divided into epitheliotropic (affinity for the epidermis, but not necessarily confined to this site), and non-epitheliotropic
- epitheliotropic forms are usually of T-lymphocyte origin and the non-epitheliotropic forms are of B-lymphocyte origin

Non-epitheliotrophic form of primary cutaneous lymphosarcoma

Clinical features

- usually multifocal or generalized erythroderma and exfoliative dermatitis
- nodules (dermoepidermal, occasionally subcutaneous)
- plaques or ulcers may be seen
- occasionally solitary nodules
- pruritus is common
- the disease may run an acute or chronic course, with systemic signs developing if metastasis to internal organs occurs. Ocular signs (anterior uveitis, hyphema and lymphocytic infiltration of the anterior chamber) are also possible

Diagnosis

- history
- physical examination
- biopsy
- further investigation includes: complete blood counts, thoracic and abdominal radiography, ophthalmic examination and microscopic assessment of lymph node and bone marrow aspirates

Treatment

- combination chemotherapy may be tried, but the outlook is very poor and euthanasia is frequently requested
- solitary lesions may be satisfactorily treated by surgical resection or cryotherapy

Epitheliotropic forms of primary cutaneous lymphosarcoma

Mycosis fungoides-like disease, pagetoid reticulosis and Sézary syndrome are epitheliotropic forms of primary lymphosarcoma.

Mycosis fungoides-like disease

- dogs and cats, older animals
- in humans mycosis fungoides is a neoplasm of T-lymphocytes, although this has not been definitely established in the dog and cat

Clinical features

- extremely variable
- usually begins as a generalized pruritic erythematous exfoliative dermatitis
- other clinical presentations include: mucocutaneous ulceration and depigmentation, cutaneous plaques or nodules — either solitary or multiple — and ulcerative oral mucosal disease
- metastatic lymphosarcoma and death ultimately supervene, on average 4 months after diagnosis (Walton 1986)
- in two cats alopecia mucinosa has been reported (Scott 1987). Both cats presented with alopecia of the head and neck. At first biopsy specimens showed mucinous degeneration of the epidermis and outer root sheath of the hair follicle. A few months later, biopsies were typical of mycosis fungoides

Diagnosis

- history
- physical examination
- skin biopsy: epitheliotropism, Pautrier's microabscesses and the presence of 'mycosis cells' and 'Sézary or Lutzner cells' (Muller *et al.* 1989)

Treatment

- the prognosis with or without treatment is poor
- combination chemotherapy
- canine mycosis fungoides has been treated in the dog with topical nitrogen mustard (Mustargen) with successful control of the cutaneous phase, although the evidence suggests that this drug has no effect on the ultimately fatal course of the condition, and is itself a topical carcinogen

Pagetoid reticulosis

- in reported canine cases clinical signs were indistinguishable from mycosis fungoides
- internal metastasis of the neoplasm occurred with later sub-epidermal infiltration of neoplastic cells

- possibly a variant of mycosis fungoides

Sézary syndrome

- rare — only one case reported to date (in a dog)
- generalized pruritus, multiple cutaneous plaques and nodules, with lymphocytic leukaemia
- histologically indistinguishable from mycosis fungoides and considered by some to be a variant of this condition
- diagnosis requires the presence of erythroderma, lymphadenopathy and the occurrence in skin biopsy of Sézary or Lutzner cells
- the reported case did not respond to treatment and euthanasia was performed

Secondary cutaneous lymphosarcoma

- tumour dissemination from another site (alimentary thymic or multicentric) to the skin
- clinical signs are those of the primary neoplasm with pruritic (occasionally non-pruritic) nodular and ulcerative skin lesions
- treatment is as for other lymphosarcomas, with combination chemotherapy, but the outlook is poor

Primary cutaneous plasmacytoma

- rare
- reported in dogs and cats
- appears to be benign since in one series all cases responded to surgical resection (Lucke 1987)
- mostly solitary tumours with a predilection for the feet, lips and ear canals
- older dogs and springer spaniels predisposed

Secondary cutaneous plasmacytoma

- multiple myeloma with secondary skin involvement
- extremely rare

MELANOCYTIC TUMOURS

Melanoma

- dogs and cats
- common in dogs but rare in cats

• benign or malignant neoplasms which arise from melanoblasts and melanocytes
• in cats no apparent breed predisposition but in dogs more common in Scottish terriers, Boston terriers, Airedales, cocker and springer spaniels, boxers, chow-chows, Dobermann pinschers and Chihuahuas. Males also appear to be predisposed

Clinical features

• older animals (average 9 years)
• usually solitary tumours
• common sites in the dog: face, feet (Fig. 63), trunk and scrotum
• common sites in the cat: head and pinnae
• oral melanomas and those arising on the lips, eyelids, digits and scrotum are usually malignant
• melanomas from other sites are more likely to be benign
• in cats most cutaneous melanomas are malignant
• benign melanomas are small, nodular and usually pigmented structures which grow slowly
• malignant melanomas grow rapidly, ulcerate and metastasize early to the regional lymph nodes, liver and lungs

Treatment

• wide, early, radical surgical excision
• the prognosis is very poor with malignant melanomas since they do not respond to chemotherapy. With oral malignant melanomas the mean survival time post-surgical removal is only 3 months

SECONDARY SKIN NEOPLASMS

• result from invasion of skin by neoplasms of non-cutaneous tissue origin, by metastasis or direct spread (e.g. from a mammary tumour)
• these neoplasms are rare in the dog and cat

NON-NEOPLASTIC TUMOURS

Epidermoid cysts (sebaceous cysts)

• common in dogs, rare in cats
• no age, sex or breed predisposition
• dermal or subcutaneous swellings, which occur most commonly on the head, neck, trunk and proximal limbs
• they may discharge a thick grey material

• thought to be acquired lesions from either displaced fragments of epithelim or occluded pilosebaceous follicles

Treatment

• surgical excision
• none

Follicular cysts (milia)

• small (2−5 mm) cysts that tend to develop if there is an obliteration to the opening of the follicle
• white or yellow in colour, they may resemble pustules or deposits of calcium as in calcinosis cutis

Trichilemmal or pilar cysts

• dogs
• resemble epidermoid cysts but are differentiated on histo-pathological examination

Dermoid cysts

• usually congenital/hereditary lesions and are discussed elsewhere in this text (Chapter 12)

Treatment

• treatment of follicular, trichilemmal and dermoid cysts is by surgical resection
• care must be taken to avoid release of the contents of the cysts into the dermis as this will provoke a foreign-body reaction

Keratoses

• firm, elevated areas of skin associated with excessive keratin production
• there are several types

Seborrhoeic keratoses

• dogs
• single or multiple
• cause unknown

• lesions are elevated plaques or nodules with a hyperkeratotic surface

Actinic keratoses

• dogs and cats
• caused by excessive exposure to ultraviolet light
• single or multiple
• lesions may be erythematous, crusting or hyperkeratotic
• they are premalignant and may develop into invasive squamous cell carcinoma

Lichenoid keratoses

• dogs
• solitary lesions seen on the pinnae of adult dogs
• lesions are erythematous plaques or papillomas

Cutaneous horns

• dogs and cats
• firm, horn-like, up to 5 cm in length
• multiple footpad cutaneous horns in the cat may be associated with feline leukaemia virus infection
• may arise from neoplasms, from keratoses or from previously healthy skin

Treatment

• most keratoses are best treated by surgical excision or by cryosurgery

Xanthoma

• dogs and cats
• benign granulomatous lesions usually associated with abnormal plasma lipid concentration or composition
• they have been reported rarely in cases of diabetes mellitus regression occurring with control of the diabetes

Hygroma

• dogs
• false or acquired bursa developing in the skin over bony prominences

- trauma-induced
- large breeds predisposed
- soft, fluid-filled swelling
- occasionally becomes infected

Treatment

- drainage, and prevent recurrence by bandaging and providing soft bedding
- recurrence may occur and these cases require more extensive surgical techniques such as extirpation, with a serious risk of wound breakdown

Calcinosis cutis

- dogs
- most common cause is naturally occurring or iatrogenic hyper-adrenocorticism (pp. 71−76)
- lesions are especially common on the dorsum, axillae and groin

Calcinosis circumscripta

- dogs
- German shepherd dogs are predisposed
- lesions tend to occur over pressure points such as the elbow and tarsal joints and the phalanges. They may also occur in the tongue
- metastatic calcinosis cutis has been reported in association with chronic renal disease (Cordy, 1967). Lesions were localized to the footpads and consisted of painful, enlarged, ulcerated footpads discharging a white gritty material

Cutaneous mucinosis

- cutaneous mucinoses are a group of conditions associated with the deposition of mucin (acid polysaccharide) in the dermis and/or epithelium
- in dogs may be seen in association with hypothyroidism, auto-immune disease and mycosis fungoides
- in cats may be associated with alopecia mucinosa and mycosis fungoides
- focal cutaneous mucinosis has been seen in Dobermann pinschers (Dillberger & Altman, 1986) the lesions presenting as soft rubbery nodules on the head or leg. Treatment consisted of surgical excision of the nodules

11/Seborrhoea

- seborrhoea is a clinical term which describes various conditions that are characterized by abnormalities of keratinization and/or sebum production
- most cases are secondary, usually chronic, and the initiating causes are extremely variable
- the key to management of the seborrhoeic conditions is therefore a careful history, a detailed examination, and laboratory investigations leading to specific treatment of the underlying cause

CANINE SEBORRHOEA

Clinical classification

Seborrhoea sicca

- the skin is dry and there is markedly increased scaling
- the Irish setter, German shepherd dog, dachshund and Doberman pinscher are predisposed

Seborrhoea oleosa

- the skin is greasy to touch, probably associated with excessive lipid production
- there is usually a strong odour
- the cocker spaniel, springer spaniel and Chinese shar pei are predisposed

Seborrhoeic dermatitis

- the skin is greasy, there is excessive scale and considerable inflammation, often associated with secondary infection
- there may be pruritus
- seborrhoeic skin has been shown to have high numbers of *Staphylococcus intermedius*, favouring the development of secondary pyoderma
- the epidermal turnover is more rapid (3−4 days) than in normal skin (21 days)
- there are also abnormalities of surface lipid content in seborrhoeic skin, particularly increased free fatty acids

146

Aetiological classification

Primary idiopathic seborrhoea

- these are cases in which no cause has been found
- cocker and springer spaniels are predisposed
- this diagnosis should be made after a full investigation of the case, because the dog will require lifelong symptomatic control, without a cure

Secondary seborrhoea

- occurs in association with a large number of skin diseases — usually in their chronic state

ENDOCRINE-RELATED
- sebum production is profoundly affected by hormonal factors. Androgens and thyroxine increase sebum and glucocorticoids and oestrogen decrease it
- seborrhoea may be secondary to hypothyroidism, hyper-adrenocorticism, gonadal abnormalities, growth hormone production abnormalities, diabetes mellitus and in cases where overdosage of glucocorticoids has been given

NUTRITION-RELATED
- dietary deficiency of protein, fat, zinc, vitamin A, for example
- maldigestion or malabsorption (pancreatic, hepatic or intestinal disease)
- fat metabolism defects (fat-responsive). No detectable clinical or dietary abnormality apart from seborrhoea and there is an improvement on supplementing the diet with fat

SYSTEMIC DISEASE
- hepatic, renal or intestinal diseases may lead to seborrhoea

ECTOPARASITIC CAUSES
- these include *Cheyletiella*, *Sarcoptes scabiei*, *Demodex* and pediculosis

HYPERSENSITIVITY DISORDERS
- atopy
- food hypersensitivity
- contact hypersensitivity

AUTOIMMUNE DISORDERS
- autoimmune disorders such as the pemphigus complex may cause seborrhoea

PYODERMA
- many cases of pyoderma will result in a secondary seborrhoea; a careful history will be helpful in deciding whether the pyoderma is primary or secondary to the seborrhoea

DERMATO-   • ringworm may produce severe scaling and crusting
PHYTOSIS

NEOPLASIA   • some neoplastic conditions, for example mycosis fungoides, may produce excessive scaling

Diagnosis

• a thorough history is essential since most cases are chronic
• note the animal's diet as some poor-quality dry and semi-moist diets may predispose to seborrhoea
• further investigations should be undertaken, following the guidelines suggested in Chapter 1
• non-specific histopathological findings include hyperkeratosis, parakeratosis, acanthosis, spongiosis and a moderate upper dermal infiltrate consisting of mononuclear cells, neutrophils and plasma cells

Treatment

• establish a cause if possible and treat this
• in primary idiopathic seborrhoea, control but not cure is possible; explain this to the owner
• antiseborrhoeic shampoos are beneficial; these may be coal-tar-based or contain selenium sulphide or salicylic acid
• shampoos containing 2.5% benzoyl peroxide are also useful in some cases
• antibacterial agents are necessary when there is a secondary pyoderma
• glucocorticoids may be used where there is severe pruritus, but they may worsen bacterial infection and alter sebum production, thus contributing to seborrhoea. Use therefore with caution
• essential fatty acid supplementation (Efavet capsules, Efamol) is beneficial in some cases

FELINE SEBORRHOEA

• less common than canine seborrhoea
• possible causes include:
any systemic disease or condition which stops grooming
low-fat diet
Cheyletiella
lice
dermatophytosis
liver disease

feline leukaemia virus infection
autoimmune disease
diabetes mellitus
hyperthyroidism
- clinically most cases present as seborrhoea sicca, but seborrhoea oleosa tends to be associated with chronic liver conditions

Treatment

- establish the cause if possible and treat specifically
- washes with selenium sulphide shampoos may be beneficial (care should be taken to rinse out the shampoo thoroughly)
- essential fatty acid supplementation (Efavet drops, Efamol) is valuable in many cases

OTHER SEBORRHOEIC SYNDROMES

Schnauzer comedo syndrome

- miniature schnauzers
- ? inherited defect
- abnormal keratinization of hair follicles
- lesions occur principally along the dorsum and consist of comedones (blackheads)
- pustule formation may follow, with associated pruritus

Diagnosis

- history
- physical examination
- biopsy — dilated hair follicles containing keratin, dilated sebaceous or apocrine glands and folliculitis

Differential diagnosis

- primary idiopathic seborrhoea
- demodicosis
- dermatophytosis
- bacterial folliculitis
- flea-bite hypersensitivity
- calcinosis cutis

Treatment

- 2.5% benzoyl peroxide shampoo as necessary

• isotretinoin (13-*cis*-retinoic acid, Accutane, Roche) at 1−2 mg/kg s.i.d. orally has proved beneficial in some cases. This drug is not licensed for the dog and is expensive. At present it is only obtainable on a named-patient basis through a consultant dermatologist

Tail gland hyperplasia

• dogs have an area on the dorsum of the tail near the base which is rich in sebaceous glands
• this area is called the supracaudal or tail gland
• in generalized seborrhoea and in conditions associated with elevated blood androgen levels, e.g. some testicular tumours, the sebaceous glands of the tail may undergo hyperplasia with an accumulation of scale and lipid. The condition is called tail gland hyperplasia or sometimes supracaudal gland seborrhoea (Fig. 64)
• usually hair is lost from the area as a result of friction and an oval area of alopecia develops
• occasionally the site is subject to secondary infection

Treatment

• if the condition is not worrying the dog do nothing except to reassure the owner
• daily antiseborrhoeic washes are helpful in more advanced cases
• castration in severe cases; surgical removal of the lesion (risk of wound breakdown)
• if part of a more generalized seborrhoeic state, further investigation of this is required

Stud tail

• most commonly, but not always, seen in entire male cats in catteries — hence the name
• in cats there is an area in the tail rich in sebaceous glands similar to the situation in the dog, but in a diffuse line along the tail
• in some cats abnormal sebaceous secretions accumulate along the dorsum of the tail, causing matting and crusting: the reason for this is not known

Treatment

• local applications of antiseborrhoeic shampoos, e.g. 2.5% benzoyl peroxide shampoo and grooming
• allow the cat free access to the outside

• progestational compounds may help, but only consider their use in severe cases, due to the possibility of undesirable side-effects
• castration is of *no* benefit

Ear margin dermatosis

• seen in middle- and old-aged dogs, especially dachshunds and other breeds with pendulous ears
• greasy tufts develop along the margins of the ears
• the tufts can be easily detached leaving a ragged margin which does not bleed
• the condition is not normally pruritic but there may occasionally be ulceration and necrosis
• partial alopecia of the pinna is noted in some cases

Treatment

• topical applications of 2.5% benzoyl peroxide shampoo
• topical application of 1% hydrocortisone cream
• control but not cure is possible

12/Congenital and Hereditary Skin Disease

Congenital conditions are present at birth. Not all are hereditary as they may occur due to an influencing factor during gestation. Other hereditary conditions may be tardive, i.e. not evident at birth but developing subsequently. Many of the conditions have been reported in small numbers; thus there is no detailed understanding of their hereditability. In most of the conditions, the animals should not be used for breeding.

Congenital alopecia

- a number of breeds have been selected for alopecia
- these include: Abyssinian dog, African sand dog, Turkish naked dog and the Peruvian hairless dog
- congenital alopecia has been reported in the miniature poodle, cocker spaniel, Belgian shepherd dog, whippet, beagle, bichon frise, basset-hound and Labrador retriever
- in some cases there is also abnormal dentition
- the sphinx cat is an example of a naturally occurring generalized alopecia
- cases of hereditary hypotrichosis have been reported in the Siamese and the Devon rex cat

Black hair follicular dysplasia

- rare
- dogs
- reported in the bearded collie, dachshund, schipperke, papillon, basset-hound and in black and white crossbreeds
- tardive

Clinical features

- affected pups are normal at birth but the defect is apparent by 4 weeks of age
- on the black parts of the coat hair fails to grow and they fracture and fall out; there is also increased scale
- the white parts of the coat are unaffected

Diagnosis

- history
- physical examination
- biopsy: histological findings include distorted hair follicles with keratinous blocking of the follicle canal

Treatment

- no treatment is effective for the follicle dysplasia
- antiseborrhoeic shampoos such as 1% selenium sulphide or 2.5% benzoyl peroxide will help control the increased scale

Colour mutant alopecia (blue Dobermann syndrome, fawn Irish setter syndrome, blue dog disease)

- one of the more common inherited canine alopecias
- breeds predisposed include: the blue Dobermann, the red and fawn Dobermann, the blue Great Dane, the blue dachshund, the blue standard poodle, the blue whippet, the blue chow-chow and the fawn Irish setter

Clinical features

- at birth the coat is normal
- a patchy 'moth-eaten' alopecia develops within the first year of life or occasionally (in Dobermanns) within the first 3 years, in the blue areas of the coat (Fig. 65)
- later there may be papules and gradual hair loss, so that after a few years most of the hair on the trunk in particular is lost
- the head, legs and the tail are spared

Diagnosis

- history
- physical examination
- elimination of other diseases
- skin biopsy: cystic hair follicles filled with keratin

Differential diagnosis

- seborrhoea complex
- dermatophytosis
- bacterial folliculitis
- demodicosis
- hypothyroidism and zinc-responsive dermatosis

Treatment

- none
- antiseborrhoeic shampoos such as 2.5% benzoyl peroxide may help the scaling

Pattern alopecia

- seen in dachshunds
- bilateral alopecia of the pinnae (males); complete by middle age
- ventral alopecia (females)
- does not respond to treatment

Melanoderma and alopecia of Yorkshire terriers

- inherited but poorly understood
- Yorkshire terriers of either sex are affected
- tardive — seen between 6 months and 3 years

Clinical features

- alopecia and hyperpigmentation
- sites affected are the bridge of the nose, the pinnae and occasionally the feet

Treatment

- none
- a few dogs spontaneously recover

CONGENITAL PIGMENTATION DEFECTS

Hereditary vitiligo

- described in the German shepherd dog, Belgian shepherd dog, Rottweiler, Dobermann pinscher, Old English sheepdog and dachshund
- hypopigmentation, especially the nose, lips, buccal mucosa, facial skin, footpads and nails

Diagnosis

- history
- physical examination
- biopsy: absence of dermal melanocytes and melanin

Treatment

- none

Canine cyclic haematopoiesis (grey collie syndrome)

- collie dogs
- puppies with the condition are born with a silver-grey coat (normal colour is sable or tricolour)
- affected puppies fail to thrive and by 6–12 weeks of age there is pyrexia, lymphadenopathy, arthralgia and diarrhoea

Diagnosis

- history
- physical examination
- laboratory investigation; there is characteristically an intermittent neutropenia alternating with neutrophilia, which continues at 10–12 day intervals. A non-regenerative anaemia ensues which is fatal

Treatment

- there is no effective treatment and once the diagnosis is established euthanasia should be advised

Tyrosinase deficiency in the chow-chow

- puppies are affected
- the normal black tongue turns pink
- occasionally the buccal mucosa is affected and hair shafts may turn white
- the condition is due to a deficiency of tyrosinase, an enzyme necessary for the synthesis of melanin

Treatment

- there is no effective treatment
- spontaneous recovery usually occurs within 2–4 months

Lentiginosis profusa

- an inherited form of melanotic macules (Briggs 1985)
- pugs
- possibly autosomal dominant mode of inheritance

Diagnosis

- history
- physical examination
- biopsy: necessary to distinguish from melanoma

Treatment

- none
- malignant transformation has not been reported in the dog

ABNORMALITIES OF STRUCTURAL INTEGRITY

Aplasia cutis (epitheliogenesis imperfecta)

- dogs and cats
- congenital discontinuity of squamous epithelium
- mode of inheritance unknown
- there is focal absence of epithelium and ulcers rapidly develop
- if the affected area is large, death results rapidly from septicaemia
- small areas may heal, and larger areas may be treatable by skin grafting, although such cases should be neutered

Cutaneous asthenia (Ehlers–Danlos syndrome, dermatosparaxis)

- dogs and cats
- inherited disorder of connective tissue
- probably inherited as an autosomal dominant trait
- breeds reported include: beagle, dachshund, boxer, St Bernard, German shepherd dog, English springer spaniel, greyhound, cross-breeds, Himalayan cat and domestic shorthair cat

Clinical features

- the skin feels soft and velvet-like
- stretching of the skin to extreme lengths is possible (Fig. 66)
- tearing of the skin is easily accomplished, and there may be multiple scars from previous traumas
- fresh wounds tend not to haemorrhage even though they are frequently considerable in size
- in man, associated abnormalities include joint hypermobility, peripheral vascular fragility, cardiac valve defects, ocular disease, bone disease and hernias

• only skin defects are noticed in the dog and cat, although lens luxation, cataract and corneal oedema, and joint laxity have been described in one dog (Barnett and Cottrell 1988)

Diagnosis

• history
• physical examination
• cutaneous biopsy: fragmented, disorganized fibrils of collagen bundles. Occasionally these are normal, and definitive diagnosis may require electron microscopical examination and biochemical studies of collagen metabolism
• extensibility index: a clinical measurement. A fold of skin is lifted up on the dorsal lumbar surface to its maximum height without causing pain. The formula used for calculating the extensibility index is:

$$\text{Extensibility index (\%)} = \frac{\text{vertical height of skin fold} \times 100}{\text{body length (occipital crest to tail base)}}$$

• affected dogs have a skin extensibility index of more than 14.5%

Treatment

• there is no treatment
• the animal should not be used for breeding
• dogs are best exercised on a lead and care taken to avoid trauma. Cats should be kept inside
• any wounds which occur are sutured promptly, using mattress sutures. Healing is usually uneventful, although owners may be discouraged if the episodes are too frequent, and request euthanasia

Dermatomyositis

• dogs
• rough collies, Shetland sheepdogs and their crosses
• breeding trials (Kunkle et al. 1985) suggest a dominant mode of inheritance with variable expression

Clinical features

• onset usually at about 3 months of age
• lesions occur around the nose, eyes, tips of the pinnae, tips of the tail and over bony prominences of the feet, elbows, stifles and sternum. Occasionally there is mucous membrane involvement
• lesions consist of papules, vesicles and pustules which later

(3—21 days) develop into crusts

• the cutaneous aspects of this condition are entirely variable: some puppies regress spontaneously early and remain in remission, while others continue with the condition until about a year of age and then go into remission with some residual focal atrophy and scarring. A few dogs persist with the problem throughout life

• there is an associated myositis which is usually not severe, and in some cases there are no detectable clinical signs. More commonly there is slight atrophy of the temporal and masseter muscles. Rarely there may be generalized atrophy of the head musculature resulting in weakness and dysphagia, and joint swelling, pyrexia and lameness

Diagnosis

• history
• physical examination
• electromyelographic (EMG) examination
• biochemical tests: plasma creatinine may be elevated
• skin biopsy: follicular atrophy and perifollicular inflammation
• muscle biopsy: myositis may be detectable in the temporal, masseter and interosseous muscles

Treatment

• not necessary in mild cases
• prednisolone (0.5 mg/kg b.i.d., reducing to alternate days) may be tried, although the efficacy is difficult to assess due to the tendency of some cases to undergo spontaneous remission
• the prognosis in most cases is favourable, with remission being usual
• affected dogs should not be bred from

MISCELLANEOUS CONDITIONS

Dermoid sinus

• dogs
• Rhodesian ridgeback (occasionally other breeds)
• incomplete dehiscence between the spinal cord and the skin during embryonic development
• possibly inherited as a simple recessive gene

Clinical features

• a small sinus is seen in the whorled hair of the dorsal cervical or sacral region

• the sinus, which is lined with epithelium, accumulates keratin and hair, and connects with the dura mater of the spinal cord

Diagnosis

• history
• physical examination

Treatment

• mild cases, none required
• more severe cases need surgical dissection

Canine icthyosis (fish-skin disease)

• congenital skin disease of dogs manifested by generalized hyperkeratosis of the skin, and with gross thickening of the digital, carpal and tarsal pads
• may be an autosomal recessive condition

Clinical features

• excessive generalized scaliness, apparent at birth, which tends to worsen with age
• the skin is covered in verrucous scales and projections of keratin material, and feels dry and rough to touch
• the pads are thickened with masses of keratin, and the foot may enlarge and become oedematous and painful

Diagnosis

• physical examination
• biopsy: marked hyperkeratosis and hypergranulosis

Differential diagnosis

• seborrhoea
• zinc-responsive dermatosis

Treatment

• incurable; advise owner of this
• antiseborrhoeic and keratolytic shampoos may help, e.g. 1% selenium sulphide (Seleen, Ceva Ltd) or 2.5% benzoyl peroxide (Oxydex, C-Vet)
• euthanasia may be requested

Epidermal dysplasia of West Highland white terriers

• thought to be an inherited disorder, although the precise mode of inheritance is unknown
• exclusively West Highland white terriers, either sex, within the first few months of age

Clinical features

• initially there is erythema and pruritus of the feet and ventrum particularly
• alopecia and hyperpigmentation develop later, and chronic cases are severely pruritic, with lichenification and seborrhoea oleosa

Diagnosis

• history
• physical examination
• biopsy: hyperplastic perivascular dermatitis with epidermal dysplasia

Differential diagnosis

• atopy
• food hypersensitivity
• flea-bite hypersensitivity
• scabies
• seborrhoea
• ichthyosis

Treatment

• some cases respond to high doses of glucocorticoids
• recently *Malassezia pachydermatis* was found to be associated with the condition as secondary overgrowth (Scott and Walton 1989) and reduction of inflammation following treatment with oral ketoconazole (Nizoral, Janssen) at a dose of 10 mg/kg daily suggests that fungal hypersensitivity is also implicated in the condition
• if there is no response to the above treatment the prognosis is poor, and many owners request euthanasia

Zinc-responsive dermatosis

• most cases seen in the UK are associated with the feeding of soya and/or cereal-based diets (see pp. 124–125)

- a hereditary defect of zinc absorption in association with chondroplasia has been described in the Alaskan malamute

Acrodermatitis

autosomal recessive trait
- described in bull-terriers
- associated with a defect in zinc metabolism

Clinical features

- lesions develop by 6 weeks of age
- the lesions are ulcerative crusts which tend to occur on the ears muzzle and feet, with keratinous projections on the footpads
- the pups are generally weak, fail to thrive and may develop respiratory infections
- most puppies die before the age of 15 months

Diagnosis

- history
- physical examination
- determination of serum zinc levels
- skin biopsy: parakeratotic hyperkeratosis

Treatment

- euthanasia should be recommended as there is no cure
- zinc supplementation does not help
- do not breed from litter mates or parents

Acral mutilation syndrome
- rare
- dogs
- English pointers and German short-haired pointers
- thought to be an autosomal recessive condition

Clinical features

- not all puppies in the litter are necessarily affected
- the lesions are first apparent between the ages of 3 and 5 months
- affected puppies begin to chew their feet
- severe mutilation occurs, yet there appears to be no pain sensation, and lameness does not occur

Diagnosis

- history
- physical examination
- histopathological examination of nerve tissue
- absence of denervation potentials on electromyographic examination

Treatment

- euthanasia should be advised and the parents of affected puppies not used for further breeding

Collagen disorder of the footpads of German shepherd dogs

- thought to be an inherited disorder
- the exact mode of inheritance has not been established

Clinical features

- German shepherd dogs of either sex
- signs first appear at between a few weeks and a few months of age
- most of the litter are affected
- the footpads, especially the carpal and tarsal pads, become soft and may ulcerate
- at this stage the puppies are healthy in all other respects

Diagnosis

- history
- physical examination
- biopsy: collagenolysis and neutrophilic inflammation

Treatment

- there is no effective treatment
- most cases regress spontaneously at 1 year of age; however, the owner must be given a very guarded prognosis since by 3 years a fatal renal amyloidosis usually develops

Digital hyperkeratosis of Irish terriers

- thought to be inherited, although the exact mode of inheritance is not understood
- very young Irish terrier puppies of either sex develop hyper-

keratosis of all footpads
- subsequently ulceration and secondary infection develop
- affected puppies are otherwise healthy

Treatment

- there is no effective cure
- excess keratin is trimmed away
- frequent warm-water bathing may help hydrate the keratin, and in conjunction petroleum jelly helps to keep the moisture in the pads
- antibacterial ointments applied daily may control the secondary infection

Lichenoid—psoriasiform dermatosis of springer spaniels

- occurs in springer spaniels of either sex at between 4 and 14 months of age
- thought to be an inherited dermatosis

Clinical features

- the lesions consist of erythematous lichenoid papules and plaques
- lesion sites tend to be pinnae, external ear canal and the inguinal region, with later spread to the rest of the face, trunk and perineum
- the lesions may become hyperkeratotic and chronic cases present as severe seborrhoea

Diagnosis

- history
- physical examination
- biopsy: lichenoid dermatitis, intraepidermal microabscesses and areas of psoriasiform epidermal hyperplasia

Treatment

- symptomatic treatment may benefit some dogs but generally there is no effective treatment

Schnauzer comedo syndrome

- exclusively miniature schnauzers
- thought to be an inherited dysplasia of hair follicles

Clinical features

- comedones develop along the dorsum
- there may also be papules and secondary folliculitis
- there are usually few symptoms, unless there is severe secondary infection

Diagnosis

- history
- physical examination
- biopsy: keratinous plugs blocking hair follicles and sebaceous gland ducts

Treatment

- most cases are controlled satisfactorily by the frequent use of 2.5% benzoyl shampoo peroxide (Oxydex, C-Vet)

Granulomatous sebaceous adenitis

- dogs
- reported in the Hungarian Vizsla, Japanese Akita, Samoyed and the black or apricot standard poodle
- thought to be inherited

Clinical features

- in certain individuals of the breeds mentioned, lesions develop along the trunk, and consist of scaling, alopecia and seborrhoea initially
- later, secondary infection frequently develops

Diagnosis

- history
- physical examination
- biopsy: granulomatous sebaceous adenitis initially, with later destruction of the sebaceous glands, a superficial perivascular dermatitis and hyperkeratosis

Differential diagnosis

- demodicosis
- dermatophytosis

- bacterial folliculitis
- endocrinopathies
- seborrhoea complex

Treatment

- the prognosis is poor in general
- symptomatic antiseborrhoea treatment may help
- isotretinoin (Accutane, Roche) at a dose of 1 mg/kg s.i.d has benefited a few dogs

13/Skin Disease of Unknown or Multiple Aetiology

Feline miliary dermatitis

- common
- any age, sex or breed

Clinical features

These are variable.
- mild papular reaction, especially on the dorsum and ventral abdomen; may not initially be noticed by the owner, but is detectable when the cat is stroked
- pruritus and self-trauma from licking
- increased fur-ball vomiting (may be the first complaint made by the owner)
- in severe cases the entire body will be affected

Causes

- flea-bite hypersensitivity; the most significant cause in areas where fleas are endemic, accounting for approximately 80% of cases. Immediate (type 1) and delayed (type 4) reactions occur to components in flea saliva
- atopy
- food hypersensitivity
- drug hypersensitivity
- intestinal parasite hypersensitivity
- feline hypereosinophilic syndrome
- *Felicola subrostratus*
- *Cheyletiella*
- *Notoedres cati*
- *Neotrombicula autumnalis*
- *Lynxacarus radovsky*
- bacterial folliculitis
- dermatophytosis
- biotin deficiency
- essential fatty acid deficiency, either dietary or secondary to maldigestion, malabsorption or liver disease
- idiopathic: should be a small percentage of cases if thorough investigation is carried out

Diagnosis

- history
- physical examination
- coat brushings, skin scrapings, fungal and bacterial culture
- dietary investigation (see food hypersensitivity, pp. 98–99)
- intradermal allergy testing (pp. 94–95)
- biopsy

Treatment

Specific treatment for an identified cause is preferable.

- initially, if fleas are suspected, a very thorough flea control programme should be carried out
- glucocorticoids: minimum dose of prednisolone to control symptoms before assessing whether flea control is proving effective
- essential fatty acid supplementation (Efavet drops, Efamol) may be a useful adjunct to treatment
- idiopathic cases may be relatively difficult to control with glucocorticoids, and in these cases there are two products which may prove to be effective:

  megesterol acetate (Ovarid, Coopers Pitman-Moore), 2.5–5 mg per cat weekly until the lesions begin to regress, then once weekly until a satisfactory response is obtained. Thereafter once-weekly maintenance doses may be given. Side-effects have been noted, including polyphagia and subsequent obesity, mammary hypertrophy, diabetes mellitus, iatrogenic Cushing's syndrome and pyometra. Most cats become more docile

  proligestone (Delvosteron, Mycofarm). 100 mg is given by subcutaneous or intramuscular injection; this may be repeated every 4 months if required

Feline indolent ulcer (eosinophilic ulcer, rodent ulcer)

- common
- may be caused by hypersensitivity reactions (atopy, food, flea-bite)

Clinical features

- either sex, more common in females, middle age
- lesions are circumscribed, glistening, ulcerative and occur mainly on the upper lip (Fig. 67)
- occasionally malignant transformation into squamous cell carcinoma may occur

• some cats have concurrent eosinophilic plaques or granulomas or both

Diagnosis

• history
• physical examination
• biopsy: non-diagnostic but differentiates from neoplasia

Treatment

• eliminate underlying cause of pruritus
• systemic glucocorticoids: prednisolone at a dose of 4.4 mg/kg s.i.d. until lesions are healed and then on alternate days
• methylprednisolone acetate injections (Depomedrone, Upjohn) at two-monthly intervals
• megestrol acetate at a dose of 5 mg twice weekly; caution is advised with this drug, as described under miliary dermatitis
• surgical removal: may be employed in selected cases but may lead to distortion of the upper lip
• other reported treatments include radiotherapy, cryotherapy, laser therapy and chrysotherapy

Feline eosinophilic plaque

• common
• cause as for indolent ulcer

Clinical features

• no age or breed predilections, females may be predisposed
• lesions may be single or multiple and consist of circumscribed, raised, red, glistening plaques
• the most common site for the lesions is the abdomen (Fig. 68) and medial thigh, but they may occur elsewhere on the skin and also in the oral cavity
• pruritus is intense

Diagnosis

• history
• physical examination
• biopsy: hyperplastic superficial and deep perivascular dermatitis with eosinophilia
• blood and tissue eosinophilia is a constant feature

Treatment

• as for indolent ulcer

Feline eosinophilic granuloma (linear granuloma)

• common
• causes as for indolent ulcer

Clinical features

• lesions may occur on the caudal thighs, on the face and in the oral cavity
• caudal thigh lesions are well circumscribed, raised, firm, glistening and linear in configuration
• lesions on the face and oral cavity are papular or nodular
• indolent ulcers or eosinophilic plaques or both may be present

Diagnosis

• history
• physical examination
• biopsy: granulomatous dermatitis with multifocal areas of collagen degeneration, foreign-body giant cells and eosinophils
• blood eosinophilia (especially oral forms)

Treatment

• as for indolent ulcer
• spontaneous regression may occur in cats less than a year of age

Canine eosinophilic granuloma

• rare
• cause is poorly understood — possibly hypersensitivity

Clinical features

• any age breed or sex, but most cases are seen at less than 3 years of age
• more common in males
• Siberian husky appears to be predisposed
• lesions are red, non-pruritic, non-painful ulcerative plaques, commonly in the oral cavity and less often on the ventral abdomen, prepuce and flanks

• occasionally lesions may occur in solitary form in the external ear canal

Diagnosis

• history
• physical examination
• biopsy: foci of collagen degeneration, infiltration of eosinophils and histiocytes, and palisading granulomas (Muller *et al.* 1989)

Treatment

• response is usually rapid (within 3 weeks) to prednisolone at a dose of 0.5−2 mg/kg/day, and permanent cure may be achieved
• some cases undergo spontaneous remission

Feline symmetric alopecia

• common
• multiple aetiology including unknown
• symmetric alopecia is preferred to the previous term endocrine alopecia, since there is no scientific proof of endocrine disorder

Clinical features

• usually in neutered males or females
• no breed predilection
• average age 6 years (range 2−12 years)
• bilaterally symmetrical hypotrichosis (not usually complete baldness), beginning in the perineal and genital regions
• later the areas affected may extend to lateral thorax and caudomedial front limbs
• there are no lesions usually and the cats are not pruritic

Diagnosis

• history
• physical examination
• elimination of other diseases presenting as alopecia
• examination of trichograms: pluck 20 or so hairs from affected areas and examine the tips under the microscope. If the tips are pointed and undamaged then the hairs are falling out and not being chewed by the cat

Differential diagnosis

- psychogenic alopecia
- demodicosis
- dermatophytosis
- flea-bite hypersensitivity
- atopy
- food hypersensitivity
- hyperadrenocorticism
- telogen and anagen defluxion

Treatment

- treat the cause if this can be diagnosed
- the idiopathic case may be treated in one of the following ways:

  thyroid hormone. Some cats with idiopathic feline symmetric alopecia may have low functional reserve (Thoday 1986), and 80% of idiopathic cases show acceptable to excellent regrowth of hair on T3 (Tertroxin, Coopers Pitman-Moore) therapy, at an initial dose of 20 μg/cat twice daily, increasing by 10 μg twice daily every third day to a maximum of 50 μg twice daily. Many cases can be satisfactorily maintained at a dose of 30 μg twice daily (Thoday 1990).

  megestrol acetate (Ovarid, Coopers Pitman-Moore) is given at a dose of 5 mg twice weekly until there is a response, then 2.5 mg once weekly. Side-effects are described under miliary dermatitis (see pp. 166–167)

  proligesterone (Delvosterone, Mycofarm) is given as an injection at a dose of 100 mg subcutaneously. This dose may be repeated in 4 months, depending on the response

  testosterone: some cases in either sex respond to an injection of testosterone (Androjet, Intervet) subcutaneously. The advised dose is 5 mg. Undesirable virilization may occur in certain individuals

  some authorities maintain that a combination of androgen/ oestrogen therapy gives better results

Feline psychogenic alopecia

- any age or sex: Siamese, Burmese or Abyssinian cats are predisposed, rare in other breeds
- may be initiated by any dermatosis, but usually caused by an 'anxiety neurosis', which is induced by any one of a variety of environmental changes upsetting the cat

Clinical features

- lesions are caused by excessive licking
- there may be alopecia with no underlying inflammation, or in chronic cases the skin may become inflamed and lichenified
- hairs at lick sites appear broken and do not epilate easily (Fig. 69)
- typical sites include the dorsum, the tail, the thighs and the ventral abdomen
- Siamese cats in particular may lick an area in the centre of the back. When the hair grows back it is darker in colour, due to the influence of temperature-labile enzymes which convert melanin precursors into melanin; the hair regains its normal colour at the next shedding

Diagnosis

- history: breed, evaluate possible psychological factors which could have initiated the problem
- physical examination
- rule out differential diagnoses

Differential diagnosis

- flea-bite hypersensitivity
- eosinophilic granuloma complex
- dermatophytosis
- demodicosis
- feline symmetric alopecia
- food hypersensitivity

Treatment

- from the history, establish a cause if possible
- glucocorticoid therapy: prednisolone on an alternate-day basis if the lesions are inflamed
- sedation: diazepam 1−2 mg b.i.d.; phenobarbitone 2−5 mg/kg b.i.d.
- megestrol acetate (Ovarid, Pitman-Moore) 2−5 mg twice weekly
- relapse occurs if the cat is psychologically upset in any way

Acral lick dermatitis ('lick granuloma')

- dogs
- Labrador and golden retriever particularly, but also the Irish

setter, German shepherd dog, Dobermann pinscher and Great Dane
• in many instances caused by psychological factors, e.g. stress or boredom, but may also occur in association with deep bacterial infection. Other factors such as bone or joint disease and hypersensitivity disorders should also be considered

Clinical features

• lesions are initially focal areas of alopecia with hyperaemia. Later erosion occurs with a sharp demarcation between normal and affected skin. They are usually solitary and commonly affect the lateral or anterior aspects of the carpus
• with chronicity, hyperpigmentation and skin-thickening occurs

Diagnosis

• history
• physical examination
• biopsy: not diagnostic in itself, but helpful to evaluate possible differential diagnoses

Differential diagnosis

• deep bacterial infection
• neoplasia
• dermatophytosis
• mycotic granulomas
• calcinosis circumscripta
• hypersensitivity disorders

Treatment

• identification and treatment where possible of underlying psychological upsets
• improve the dog's life style (more walks, less time alone, provide a companion, etc.)
• rigorous antibacterial therapy is frequently beneficial
• glucocorticoid therapy (topical, subcutaneously, intra- or sublesionally)
• surgical resection (risk of breakdown)
• cryosurgery
• radiation therapy is occasionally effective
• the prognosis for cure is guarded since lesions may heal with difficulty, or heal and be replaced by new lesions

Panniculitis (nodular panniculitis)

- dogs and cats
- multifactorial inflammatory condition of the subcutaneous fat
- may be caused by bacterial and fungal infections, autoimmune disorders, foreign bodies, vascular embolism or vitamin E deficiency, but the great majority of cases in the dog and cat are idiopathic
- any breed of dog and cat, but the dachshund may be predisposed

Clinical features

- the lesions are deep cutaneous nodules, single (more usual in cats) or multiple
- the nodules are firm and may develop draining tracts discharging an oily substance, and may ulcerate
- a few animals are systemically ill (lethargy, pyrexia)

Diagnosis

- history
- physical examination
- biopsy: a complete nodule must be excised for histopathological examination, which typically shows pyogranulomatous panniculitis

Differential diagnosis

- neoplasia
- deep pyoderma
- cysts

Treatment

- excision for solitary lesions
- glucocorticoids: prednisolone 1 mg/kg (dogs) and 2 mg/kg (cats). Remission is usually obtained within 2 weeks and many cases, especially young dogs, will remain in remission with no further treatment; other cases may require prolonged treatment on an alternate-day basis
- vitamin E (DL-α-tocopheryl acetate) 400 IU b.i.d. has been beneficial in some cases

Acanthosis nigricans

- uncommon
- dogs

- multifactorial causes: friction secondary to obesity, endocrinopathies, hypersensitivity disorders, and idiopathic
- these cases are managed by identification of the precipitating
cause and its specific treatment
- idiopathic cases are seen almost exclusively in the dachshund

Idiopathic acanthosis nigricans

- dachshunds

Clinical features

- onset usually before 1 year of age
- the initial lesion is an area of bilateral axillary hyperpigmentation
- later there is alopecia and lichenification, which in severe chronic
cases may spread to most of the body, with secondary pyoderma
and seborrhoea

Diagnosis

- history
- physical examination
- investigation of other possible causes
- biopsy is non-specific and typical of chronic inflammation
- response to treatment

Treatment

- melatonin (Rickards Research Foundation) has been used in the
USA. This drug, a pineal gland hormone, is given as a subcutaneous
injection at a dose of 2 mg per dog daily for 3–5 days, then weekly
and later monthly as required
- prednisolone given on alternate days following a loading dose of
1 mg/kg b.i.d.
- some dogs have responded to vitamin E at a dose of 400 IU orally
per day

Juvenile cellulitis (juvenile pyoderma, puppy strangles)

- dogs
- cause unknown — possibly a hypersensitivity response

Clinical features

- begins in puppies between the ages of 3 weeks to 4 months

• any breed, but dachshunds, pointers, golden retrievers and Gordon setters may be predisposed
• one or more puppies or the whole litter may develop the condition
• lesion sites are the lips, eyelids and occasionally the ears, prepuce and anus (Fig. 70)
• affected skin is hyperaemic and oedematous and oozes serum or pus, which develops honey-coloured crusts
• gross submandibular lymphadenopathy is a marked and constant feature (hence puppy strangles)
• abscessation may occur from the lymph nodes
• affected animals may be well or pyrexic and depressed

Diagnosis

• history
• physical examination
• biopsy: diffuse cellulitis
• careful sampling of intact pustules: usually sterile — occasionally *S. intermedius* is isolated

Treatment

• the cornerstone of treatment is glucocorticoids
• prednisolone is given by mouth at a dose of 1 mg/kg b.i.d.
• antibacterial drugs are given as an adjunct to therapy — alone they are ineffective
• early diagnosis and aggressive treatment are required for this condition or scarring of the skin will result

Subcorneal pustular dermatosis

• very rare
• dogs
• cause unknown

Clinical features

• any breed, age or sex; miniature schnauzers are predisposed
• lesions are initially pustules. These are non-follicular and greenish-yellow in colour, and are transient. More common subsequent lesions are circular patches of alopecia, erosions, crusts and seborrhoea
• lesion sites are the head and trunk
• pruritus may be severe or absent
• the dogs are otherwise healthy

Diagnosis

- history
- physical examination
- elimination of other diagnoses
- skin biopsy: subcorneal pustular dermatitis
- cultures from intact pustules are usually negative

Differential diagnosis

- bacterial folliculitis
- dermatophytosis
- demodicosis
- pemphigus complex
- systemic lupus erythematosus
- seborrhoea
- hypersensitivity disorders (atopy, food hypersensitivity)

Treatment

- dapsone (Avlosulfon) 1 mg/kg t.i.d.
- response usually occurs within a month; maintenance doses of 1 mg/kg s.i.d. can then be given twice weekly
- in some cases cure is achieved, no further treatment being required
- possible side-effects of dapsone include hepatotoxicity, non-regenerative anaemia and leucopenia; these usually occur early in treatment and are reversible if the treatment is stopped
- some dogs which do not respond to dapsone benefit from treatment with sulphasalazine (Salazopyrin, Pharmacia Ltd) at a dose of 10−20 mg/kg t.i.d. orally; long-term administration of this drug may induce keratoconjunctivitis sicca

14/Diseases of Ears, Eyelids and Nails

EAR DISEASES

Otitis externa

- common
- inflammation of the outer ear (otitis externa) is always associated with predisposing factors. Examples of these include:
  a long, relatively narrow ear canal
  pendulous ear flaps (89% of otitis externa involves long-eared dogs)
  hair, e.g. poodles, Yorkshire terriers
  concurrent diseases, e.g. atopy, hypothyroidism, seborrhoea, scabies, ear mites
  foreign body, e.g. grass awn
  tumours, e.g. sebaceous gland adenoma, adenocarcinoma, ceruminous gland tumour and squamous cell carcinoma
  moist environment, swimming

Pathogenesis

When one or more of these predisposing factors induces inflammation, there is hyperplasia and erythema of the ear lining. This may lead to excess wax formation, which encourages bacteria and yeasts. If the condition becomes chronic, there is restriction of the external ear lumen, leading to poor drainage. In neglected cases the tympanic membrane may rupture. Constant trauma of the pinna may lead to the development of fissures.

Common organisms isolated from the ear canal in cases of otitis externa include:
- *Staphylococcus* spp.
- *Streptococcus*
- *Escherichia coli*
- *Proteus*
- *Pseudomonas*
- the yeast *Malassezia pachydermitis*

Diagnosis

- history
- physical examination — tranquillization or light anaesthesia should

be considered if adequate examination is difficult
• culture and bacterial sensitivity are indicated in long-standing cases. Useful information may also be obtained by Diff-quik stain of exudates

Treatment

Grono (1980) has suggested a protocol for the management of otitis externa:
• sedate or anaesthetize the patient
• a swab is taken for staining and bacterial culture and sensitivity testing
• debris and discharge are removed by gently irrigating the ear with either 0.5% chlorhexidine or cetrimide
• the ear is then flushed with saline and dried
• re-examination is made with an otoscope
• pendulous ears are strapped over the head
• specific medication is applied
• treatment is changed as necessary indicated by the laboratory findings
   In general it is preferable to treat specifically and avoid, if possible, polypharmaceutical products.
   There are three broad categories of aural products available for the treatment of otitis externa:
• antibacterial and antimycotic. Many of these products have neomycin as the main antibacterial ingredient. Some also contain glucocorticoids
• acaricidal. A common ingredient in many preparations is gamma benzene hexachloride
• ear cleansing and cerumenolytic preparations
   A fourth group consists of products which attempt to treat all possibilities. These products are less desirable since it becomes difficult to assess therapeutic efficacy

Aural haematoma

• may result from flapping of the pinnae due to otitis externa
• it has recently been suggested (Kuwahara 1986) that aural haematoma may be associated with autoimmune disorders, since in many cases there were positive Coombs' tests, ANA tests and immunoglobulin deposits at the dermoepidermal junction

Treatment

• investigate and correct the underlying cause

• surgical drainage of the aural haematoma

EYELID DISEASES

Blepharitis

Blepharitis is inflammation of the eyelid margin. Causes include:
• dermatophytosis (myotic blepharitis)
• demodicosis
• staphyloccocal infection
• juvenile cellulitis
• atopy
• food hypersensitivity
• primary seborrhoea
• autoimmune disorders, e.g. pemphigus complex, bullous pemphigoid
   Diagnosis and treatment of these conditions has been discussed elsewhere in the text.

Entropion (inversion of the eyelids) and *ectropion* (eversion of the eyelids) are anatomical defects of the eyelids which lead to chronic conjunctivitis.

Trichiasis is the term used for abnormal direction of the normal eyelid cilia, which rub on the cornea, provoking inflammation and sometimes ulceration.

Distichiasis is the presence of ectopic cilia on the tarsal plate, which rub on the cornea.

In addition to corneal problems, self-trauma may induce blepharitis in the above conditions. Their management is by surgical correction of the anatomical defect, and the reader is referred to standard ophthalmological texts.

Hordeolum is the term for pyogenic infection of a sebaceous gland of the eyelid.

External hordeolum affects the outer eyelid glands of Zeiss and cilia.

Internal hordeolum (meibomian sty) affects the inner meibomian gland.

Treatment

- surgical drainage of the abscess
- topical antibacterial ointments

NAIL DISEASES

Paronychia

- inflammation of the soft tissues around the nail base
- causes include:
  bacteria
  fungi
  demodicosis
  pemphigus complex
  bullous pemphigoid
  systemic lupus erythematosus
  diabetes mellitus

Pyonychia is characterized by a purulent exudate at the base of the nail.

Treatment

- treatment should be directed at the precipitating cause if this can be found
- where no precipitating cause is found, many cases benefit from surgical removal of the nail plate followed by supportive antibacterial therapy

Onychomycosis

- fungal infection of the nail
- rare
- dogs and cats
- usually *Trichophyton mentagrophytes* is incriminated
- frequently there is nail deformity

Treatment

- surgical removal of the entire third phalanx
- long-term (several months at least) oral griseofulvin

Onychorrhexis

- brittle nails
- if single nails are involved, the most common cause is trauma
- multiple nails may be involved and the cause in these cases is unknown. There is a breed predilection for dachshunds

Treatment

- intractable cases are best treated by surgical removal of the entire nail
- warm-water soaks and trimming of splinters may afford temporary relief

Onychomadesis

- separation of the nail shell
- causes include trauma, infection and autoimmune disease
- treatment involves investigation and specific therapy of the possible underlying causes

Selected Reading

Baker, B.B. & Maibach, H.I. (1987) Epidermal cell renewal in seborrheic skin disease in dogs. *Am. J. Vet. Res.* **48**, 726.

Baker, K.P. & Thomsett, L.R. (1990) *Canine and Feline Dermatology*. Blackwell Scientific Publication, Oxford.

Barnett, K.C. & Cottrell, B.D. (1988) Ehlers–Danlos syndrome in a dog: ocular, cutaneous and articular abnormalities. *J. Small Anim. Pract.* **28**, 941.

Barta, O., Waltmann, C., Oyekan, P.P. *et al.* (1983) Lymphocyte transformation suppression caused by pyoderma — failure to demonstrate it in uncomplicated demodectic mange. *Comp. Immunol. Microbiol. Infect. Dis.* **6**, 9.

Bevier, D.E. & Goldschmidt, M.H. (1981) Skin tumours in the dog. Part I. Epithelial tumours and tumour-like lesions. *Comp. Cont. Ed. Small Anim. Pract.* **3**, 389.

Bevier, D.E. & Goldschmidt, M.H. (1981) Skin tumours in the dog. Part II. Tumours of the soft (mesenchymal) tissues. *Comp. Cont. Ed. Small Anim. Pract.* **3**, 506.

Briggs, O.M. (1985) Lentiginosis profusa in the pug: three case reports. *J. Small Anim. Pract.* **26**, 675.

Cordy, D.R. (1967) Apocrine cystic calcinosis in dogs and its relationship to chronic renal disease. *Cornell Vet.* **57**, 107.

Dillberger, J.E. & Altman, N.H. (1986) Focal mucinosis in dogs. Seven cases of a review of cutaneous mucinoses of man and animals. *Vet. Pathol.* **23**, 132.

Grono, L.R. (1980) Otitis externa. In *Current Veterinary Therapy VII* (ed. R.W. Kirk), Saunders, Philadelphia, p. 403.

Halliwell, R.E.W. & Gorman N.T. (1989) In *Veterinary Clinical Immunology*. Saunders, Philadelphia.

Halliwell, R.E.W. & Werner, L.L. (1979) Autoimmune disease. In *Canine Medicine and Therapeutics* (eds E.A. Chandler *et al.*), Blackwell Scientific Publications, Oxford, p. 24.

Halliwell, R.E.W., Preston, J.F. & Nesbitt, J.G. (1987) Aspects of the immunopathogenesis of flea allergic dermatitis in dogs. *Vet. Immunol. Immunopathol.* **15**, 203.

Herrtage, M.E. (1990) The adrenal gland. In *Manual of Small Animal Endocrinology* (ed. M.F. Hutchinson), B.S.A.V.A., Cheltenham.

Ihrke, P.J. (1983) The management of canine pyodermas. In *Current Veterinary Therapy VIII* (ed. R.W. Kirk), Saunders, Philadelphia, p. 505.

Ihrke, P.J. (1987) An overview of bacterial skin disease in the dog. *Br. Vet. J.* **143**, 112.

Ihrke, P.J. & Goldschmidt, M.H. (1983) Vitamin A-responsive dermatosis in the cocker spaniel. *J. Am. Vet. Med. Assoc.* **188**, 877.

Kunkle, G.A. (1980) Zinc-responsive dermatosis in dogs. In *Current Veterinary Therapy VII* (ed. R.W. Kirk), Saunders, Philadelphia, p. 472.

Kunkle, G.A. (1981) Managing canine seborrhea. In *Current Veterinary Therapy VIII* (ed. R.W. Kirk), Saunders, Philadelphia, p. 516.

Kunkle, G.A., Gross, T.L. & Fadok, V. (1985) Dermatomyositis in Collie dogs. *Comp. Cont. Ed. Pract. Vet.* **7**, 3, 185.

Kuwahara, J. (1986) Canine and feline aural hematoma: clinical, experimental and clinicopathologic observation. *Am. J. Vet. Res.* **47**, 2300.

Larsson, M. (1988) Determination of free thyroxine and cholesterol as a new screening test of canine hypothyroidism. *J. Am. Anim. Hosp. Assoc.* **24**, 209.

Longstaffe, J.A. & Guy, M.W. (1985) Leishmaniasis in dogs. *Vet. Ann.* **25**, 358.

Lloyd, D.H. (1985) Diagnosis methods in dermatology. *Br. Vet. J.* **141**, 463.

Lucke, V.R. (1987) Primary cutaneous plasmacytoma in the dog and cat. *J. Small Anim. Pract.* **28**, 49.

Macey, D.W. & Reynolds, H.A. (1981) The incidence, characterisation and clinical management of skin tumors of cats. *J. Am. Anim. Hosp. Assoc.* **17** (6), 1026.

McCartney, L., Ryecroft, A.W. & Hammil, L. (1988) Cutaneous prototheceosis in the dog: first confirmed case in Britain. *Vet. Rec.* **123** (19), 494.

Muller, G.H., Kirk, R.W. & Scott, D.W. (1989) In *Small Animal Dermatology*, 4th edn. W.B. Saunders, Philadelphia.

Nesbitt, G.H. (1983) In *Canine and Feline Dermatology: A Systematic Approach*. Lea & Febiger, Philadelphia.

Peterson, M.E., Krieger, D.T. Drucker, W.D. *et al.* (1982) Immunocytochemical study of the hypophysis in 25 dogs with pituitary-dependent hyperadrenocorticism. *Acta Endocrinol.* **101**, 15.

Reedy, L.M. & Muller, W.H. (1989) *Allergic Skin Disease of Dogs and Cats.* Saunders, Philadelphia.

Scott, D.W. (1987) Feline dermatology 1983–1985: 'the secret sits'. *J. Am. Anim. Hosp. Assoc.* **23**, 255.

Scott, D.W. & Muller, W.H. (1989) Epidermal dysplasia and *Malassezia pachydermatis* infection in West Highland white terriers. *Vet. Dermatol.* **1**, 25.

Scott, D.W., Schultz, R.D. & Baker, E. (1976) Further studies on the therapeutic and immunologic aspects of generalised demodectic mange in the dog. *J. Am. Anim. Hosp. Assoc.* **12**, 203.

Scott, D.W., Walton, D.K., Slater, M.R. *et al.* (1987) Immune-mediated dermatoses in domestic animals: ten years after. Part I. *Comp. Cont. Ed. Pract. Vet.* **9**, 4, 424.

Tams, T.R. & Macy, D.W. (1981) Canine mast cell tumours. *Comp. Cont. Ed. Pract. Vet.* **3**, 869.

Thoday, K.L. (1981) Investigative techniques in small animal dermatology. *Br. Vet. J.* **137**, 133.

Thoday, K.L. (1986) The differential diagnosis of symmetric alopecia in the cat. In *Current Veterinary Therapy IX* (ed. R.W. Kirk), Saunders, Philadelphia, p. 545.

Thoday, K.L. (1989) Diet-related zinc-responsive skin disease in dogs: a dying dermatosis? *J. Small Anim. Pract.* **30**, 213.

Thoday, K.L. (1990) The thyroid gland. In *Manual of Small Animal Endocrinology* (ed. M.F. Hutchinson), B.S.A.V.A., Cheltenham.

Walton, D.K. (1986) Canine epidermotropic lymphoma (mycosis fungoides and pagetoid reticulosis). In *Current Veterinary Therapy IX* (ed. R.W. Kirk), Saunders, Philadelphia, p. 609.

Walton, D.K., Center, S.A., Scott, D.W. *et al.* (1986) Ulcerative dermatosis associated with diabetes mellitus in the dog: a report of 4 cases. *J. Am. Anim. Hosp. Assoc.* **22** (1), 79.

Walton, G.S. (1977) Allergic contact dermatitis. In *Current Veterinary Therapy VI* (ed. R.W. Kirk), Saunders, Philadelphia, p. 571.

Willemse, T.A. (1986) Atopic dermatitis. In *Dermatology* (ed. G.H. Nesbitt), Churchill Livingstone, New York, p. 57.

Willemse, T.A., Van den Brom, W.E. & Rijnberg, A. (1984) Effect of hyposensitization on atopic dermatitis in dogs. *J. Am. Vet. Med. Assoc.* **184**, 1277.

Wright, A.I. (1989) Ringworm in dogs and cats. *J. Small Anim. Pract.* **30**, 242.

Index